small animal
internal medicine
case management
test booklet

The National Veterinary Medical Series for Independent Study

small animal internal medicine case management test booklet

Darcy H. Shaw, D.V.M., M.V.Sc
Diplomate ACVIM (Internal Medicine)
Associate Professor
Department of Companion Animals
University of Prince Edward Island
Charlottetown, Prince Edward Island, Canada

Sherri L. Ihle, D.V.M., M.V.Sc
Diplomate ACVIM (Internal Medicine)
Associate Professor
Department of Companion Animals
University of Prince Edward Island
Charlottetown, Prince Edward Island, Canada

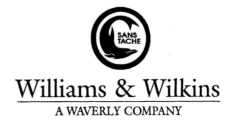

Williams & Wilkins
A WAVERLY COMPANY

BALTIMORE • PHILADELPHIA • LONDON • PARIS • BANGKOK
BUENOS AIRES • HONG KONG • MUNICH • SYDNEY • TOKYO • WROCLAW

1997

Editor: Elizabeth Nieginski
Manager, Development Editor: Julie A. Scardiglia
Managing Editor: Darrin Kiessing
Marketing Manager: Diane M. Harnish
Production Coordinator: Cindy Park
Design Coordinator: Mario Fernandez
Typesetter: Port City Press, Inc.
Printer: The Mack Printing Group
Digitized Illustrations: Port City Press, Inc.
Binder: The Mack Printing Group

351 West Camden Street
Baltimore, Maryland 21201-2436 USA

Rose Tree Corporate Center
1400 North Providence Road
Building II, Suite 5025
Media, Pennsylvania 19063-2043 USA

Accurate indications, adverse reactions and dosage schedules for drugs are provided in this book, but it is possible that they may change. The reader is urged to review the package information data of the manufacturers of the medications mentioned.

First Edition

Library of Congress Cataloging-in-Publication Data

Shaw, Darcy H.
    Small animal internal medicine case management test booklet / Darcy H. Shaw, Sherri L. Ihle.
      p.   cm. — (The National veterinary medical series for independent study)
    ISBN 0-683-30348-1
    1. Dogs—Diseases. 2. Cats—Diseases. 3. Veterinary internal medicine. I. Ihle, Sherri L.
II. Title. III. Series.
SF991.S534 1997   97-8339
636.7′0896—dc21   CIP

The Publishers have made every effort to trace the copyright holders for borrowed material. If they have inadvertently overlooked any, they will be pleased to make the necessary arrangements at the first opportunity.

To purchase additional copies of this book, call our customer service department at **(800) 638-0672** or fax orders to **(800) 447-8438.** For other book services, including chapter reprints and large quantity sales, ask for the Special Sales department.

Canadian customers should call **(800) 665-1148,** or fax **(800) 665-0103.** For all other calls originating outside of the United States, please call **(410) 528-4223** or fax us at **(410) 528-8550.**

Visit Williams & Wilkins on the Internet: **http://www.wwilkins.com** or contact our customer service department at **custserv@wwilkins.com.** Williams & Wilkins customer service representatives are available from 8:30 am to 6:00 pm, EST, Monday through Friday, for telephone access.

97 98 99 00
1 2 3 4 5 6 7 8 9 10

Dedication

To my grandmother, Margaret Lerner, whose patience, pragmatism, and delectable strudel made growing up just a little bit easier.

To my parents, Rose and Harold Shaw, for their love and support.

D.H.S.

Contents

Preface

The objective of *NVMS Small Animal Internal Medicine—Case Management Test Booklet* is to provide the reader with the opportunity to apply medical knowledge in the diagnosis and treatment of disease. Twelve cases are presented. The reader is provided with the signalment and presenting complaint. Following this, additional information can be sought for historical and physical examination findings. Next, the reader can choose from an extensive list of diagnostic tests to reach a final diagnosis. Finally, a treatment plan is selected and the response to treatment can then be looked up. A discussion of the optimal diagnostic approach, diagnosis, and the most appropriate treatment is provided for each case.

The design of the cases is meant to simulate real case management and is also very similar to the method employed in the clinical competency portion of national board examinations. Approximate costs for diagnostic tests and procedures are included. Although costs are not a feature of board examinations, they will encourage the reader to select diagnostic tests in an efficient manner that reflects the realities of clinical practice. The case management exercises will be very useful to third- and fourth-year veterinary students, as well as to interns and practitioners.

We expect that the reader will find the cases challenging and intriguing. Good luck!

Darcy H. Shaw
Sherri L. Ihle

Acknowledgments

The authors would like to thank Elizabeth Nieginski for her ideas and support, Darrin Kiessling for his editorial contributions, and Cindy Park for her work in production.

Section I

Opening Scenarios

Directions: Each of the following patient management problems is based on an actual clinical case. Follow the instructions found at the beginning of each part. A summary of the optimal diagnostic approach, diagnosis, and treatment for each case is located at the end of the text.

Case 1. A 5-year-old male neutered Doberman pinscher weighing 37 kg (82 lbs) is presented because of episodes of weakness.

Case 2. An 11-year-old male neutered mixed-breed dog weighing 11 kg (24 lbs) is presented because of acute collapse.

Case 3. A 6-year-old female spayed Newfoundland weighing 56 kg (124 lbs) is presented because of epistaxis.

Case 4. A 2.5-year-old female domestic shorthair cat weighing 3.4 kg (7.5 lbs) is presented because of dyspnea.

Case 5. A 3-year-old female miniature dachshund weighing 5.6 kg (12.3 lbs) is presented because of coughing.

Case 6. A 2-year-old male neutered mixed-breed dog weighing 27 kg (60 lbs) is presented because of depression and ataxia.

Case 7. A 9-year-old female miniature poodle weighing 7 kg (15.4 lbs) is presented because of increased urination.

Case 8. A 6-year-old male neutered German shepherd dog weighing 34 kg (75 lbs) is presented because of increased urination and hematuria.

Case 9. A 4-year-old female spayed mixed-breed dog weighing 9 kg (20 lbs) is presented because of intermittent diarrhea.

Case 10. A 1-year-old female spayed Great Dane weighing 50 kg (110 lbs) is presented because of anorexia and weakness.

Case 11. A 14-month-old female miniature schnauzer weighing 8 kg (17.6 lbs) is presented because of seizures.

Case 12. A 7-year-old female golden retriever weighing 33 kg (72.6 lbs) is presented because of vomiting and lethargy.

1

Parts A and B
History and Physical
Examination

Directions: Select the additional history you desire and look up the corresponding number in the *Answers for Parts A and B (History and Physical Examination).* After you have obtained all your desired history, go to Part B.

To avoid bias and to make the case management exercise as realistic as possible, please read only the selected numbered answer.

Onset and duration of the current problem

Case 1=198	Case 2=89	Case 3=37	Case 4=69	Case 5=103	Case 6=184
Case 7=176	Case 8=1	Case 9=164	Case 10=146	Case 11=126	Case 12=81

Specific signs observed in relation to the current problem

Case 1=82	Case 2=104	Case 3=186	Case 4=147	Case 5=199	Case 6=2
Case 7=127	Case 8=38	Case 9=70	Case 10=165	Case 11=181	Case 12=177

Progression of the current signs

Case 1=182	Case 2=71	Case 3=39	Case 4=200	Case 5=166	Case 6=178
Case 7=206	Case 8=148	Case 9=83	Case 10=105	Case 11=3	Case 12=128

Current or recent treatments for the problem

Case 1=40	Case 2=40	Case 3=40	Case 4=40	Case 5=40	Case 6=40
Case 7=40	Case 8=40	Case 9=4	Case 10=40	Case 11=40	Case 12=40

Ownership history

Case 1=41	Case 2=5	Case 3=41	Case 4=106	Case 5=41	Case 6=72
Case 7=41	Case 8=41	Case 9=41	Case 10=41	Case 11=41	Case 12=41

Vaccination history

Case 1=6	Case 2=42	Case 3=107	Case 4=129	Case 5=6	Case 6=42
Case 7=73	Case 8=149	Case 9=149	Case 10=167	Case 11=149	Case 12=167

Past medical history

Case 1=201	Case 2=108	Case 3=168	Case 4=84	Case 5=7	Case 6=74
Case 7=150	Case 8=43	Case 9=130	Case 10=130	Case 11=74	Case 12=179

Travel history, place of residence

Case 1=169	Case 2=131	Case 3=109	Case 4=44	Case 5=180	Case 6=8
Case 7=202	Case 8=187	Case 9=75	Case 10=75	Case 11=151	Case 12=85

Breeding history

Case 1=9	Case 2=110	Case 3=132	Case 4=152	Case 5=170	Case 6=9
Case 7=45	Case 8=76	Case 9=132	Case 10=132	Case 11=152	Case 12=190

Current medication(s)

Case 1=46	Case 2=46	Case 3=46	Case 4=77	Case 5=46	Case 6=46
Case 7=46	Case 8=10	Case 9=10	Case 10=10	Case 11=10	Case 12=10

Historical adverse drug reactions

Case 1=11	Case 2=11	Case 3=11	Case 4=11	Case 5=11	Case 6=11
Case 7=11	Case 8=11	Case 9=11	Case 10=11	Case 11=11	Case 12=11

Diet type, amount, and feeding schedule

Case 1=47	Case 2=78	Case 3=203	Case 4=191	Case 5=12	Case 6=47
Case 7=171	Case 8=133	Case 9=12	Case 10=153	Case 11=111	Case 12=47

Housing/general environment

Case 1=79	Case 2=79	Case 3=134	Case 4=13	Case 5=154	Case 6=134
Case 7=48	Case 8=112	Case 9=79	Case 10=172	Case 11=48	Case 12=79

Exposure to other animals

Case 1=173	Case 2=14	Case 3=80	Case 4=192	Case 5=204	Case 6=80
Case 7=155	Case 8=113	Case 9=14	Case 10=49	Case 11=14	Case 12=135

Appetite

Case 1=50	Case 2=15	Case 3=50	Case 4=114	Case 5=50	Case 6=136
Case 7=50	Case 8=50	Case 9=193	Case 10=90	Case 11=156	Case 12=174

Water intake

Case 1=137	Case 2=175	Case 3=157	Case 4=205	Case 5=16	Case 6=51
Case 7=194	Case 8=91	Case 9=16	Case 10=16	Case 11=16	Case 12=115

Urination/defecation habits

Case 1=158	Case 2=158	Case 3=158	Case 4=158	Case 5=158	Case 6=158
Case 7=17	Case 8=116	Case 9=52	Case 10=92	Case 11=158	Case 12=158

Other clinical signs or changes noted

Case 1=117	Case 2=53	Case 3=139	Case 4=139	Case 5=139	Case 6=139
Case 7=139	Case 8=139	Case 9=18	Case 10=139	Case 11=93	Case 12=208

PART B **Directions:** Select the physical examination results you desire and look up the corresponding number in the *Answers for Parts A and B (History and Physical Examination).* When you have obtained all your desired physical examination results, go to Part C.

General appearance

Case 1=195	Case 2=118	Case 3=54	Case 4=183	Case 5=54	Case 6=86
Case 7=185	Case 8=94	Case 9=140	Case 10=159	Case 11=19	Case 12=188

Locomotion

Case 1=141	Case 2=119	Case 3=141	Case 4=141	Case 5=141	Case 6=20
Case 7=141	Case 8=141	Case 9=141	Case 10=56	Case 11=141	Case 12=95

Temperature

Case 1=21	Case 2=160	Case 3=21	Case 4=196	Case 5=57	Case 6=120
Case 7=21	Case 8=57	Case 9=57	Case 10=96	Case 11=21	Case 12=142

Pulse rate

Case 1=189	Case 2=97	Case 3=197	Case 4=22	Case 5=87	Case 6=143
Case 7=58	Case 8=121	Case 9=58	Case 10=161	Case 11=58	Case 12=121

Respiratory rate

Case 1=23	Case 2=59	Case 3=59	Case 4=162	Case 5=144	Case 6=122
Case 7=98	Case 8=23	Case 9=98	Case 10=23	Case 11=98	Case 12=23

Ocular examination

Case 1=60	Case 2=60	Case 3=60	Case 4=60	Case 5=60	Case 6=24
Case 7=60	Case 8=60	Case 9=60	Case 10=60	Case 11=60	Case 12=60

Oral examination, mucous membrane color, capillary refill time

Case 1=123	Case 2=207	Case 3=61	Case 4=123	Case 5=123	Case 6=123
Case 7=123	Case 8=123	Case 9=123	Case 10=25	Case 11=123	Case 12=99

Otic examination

Case 1=62	Case 2=62	Case 3=100	Case 4=62	Case 5=62	Case 6=62
Case 7=26	Case 8=62	Case 9=62	Case 10=62	Case 11=62	Case 12=62

Head and neck symmetry

Case 1=27	Case 2=27	Case 3=27	Case 4=27	Case 5=27	Case 6=27
Case 7=27	Case 8=27	Case 9=27	Case 10=27	Case 11=27	Case 12=27

Larynx/trachea palpation

Case 1=63	Case 2=63	Case 3=63	Case 4=63	Case 5=28	Case 9=63
Case 7=63	Case 8=63	Case 9=63	Case 10=63	Case 11=63	Case 12=63

Lymph node palpation

Case 1=29	Case 2=29	Case 3=29	Case 4=29	Case 5=29	Case 6=64
Case 7=29	Case 8=29	Case 9=29	Case 10=29	Case 11=29	Case 12=29

Palpation of thorax

Case 1=30	Case 2=30	Case 3=30	Case 4=65	Case 5=30	Case 6=30
Case 7=30	Case 8=30	Case 9=30	Case 10=30	Case 11=30	Case 12=30

Thoracic auscultation

Case 1=31	Case 2=145	Case 3=31	Case 4=101	Case 5=66	Case 6=31
Case 7=31	Case 8=31	Case 9=31	Case 10=124	Case 11=31	Case 12=31

Abdominal palpation

Case 1=125	Case 2=32	Case 3=125	Case 4=125	Case 5=125	Case 6=125
Case 7=163	Case 8=67	Case 9=102	Case 10=125	Case 11=125	Case 12=88

Genitalia

Case 1=68	Case 2=68	Case 3=33	Case 4=33	Case 5=33	Case 6=68
Case 7=33	Case 8=68	Case 9=33	Case 10=33	Case 11=33	Case 12=33

Skin/mammary glands

Case 1=34	Case 2=34	Case 3=34	Case 4=34	Case 5=34	Case 6=34
Case 7=34	Case 8=34	Case 9=34	Case 10=34	Case 11=34	Case 12=34

Limbs

Case 1=35	Case 2=35	Case 3=35	Case 4=35	Case 5=35	Case 6=35
Case 7=35	Case 8=35	Case 9=35	Case 10=35	Case 11=35	Case 12=35

Anus/tail

Case 1=36	Case 2=36	Case 3=36	Case 4=36	Case 5=36	Case 6=36
Case 7=36	Case 8=36	Case 9=36	Case 10=36	Case 11=36	Case 12=36

Answers for Parts A and B
(History and Physical Examination)

PARTS A & B

1. The problem was first noticed 3 to 4 weeks ago. The owners did not bring the dog in sooner because they thought the problem might resolve without treatment.

2. The owner describes the dog as being disinterested in its surroundings, having difficulty rising, lacking coordination, and holding its neck extended.

3. The first seizure was seen 4 months ago. Subsequently, no seizures occurred for 3 months, but in the last month two seizures have been observed.

4. Previous treatment with oral amoxicillin and fenbendazole had no effect.

5. The dog has been owned by the current owners since it was 2 years of age.

6. The last vaccination was given 14 months ago and included distemper virus, parainfluenza, adenovirus-2, parvovirus, coronavirus, and rabies.

7. The dog had superficial pyoderma that was successfully treated 2 years previously, and had a litter of 3 healthy puppies 4 months ago.

8. The dog resides in Indiana and has never left the area.

9. The dog was neutered at 7 months of age.

10. The dog has received ivermectin as heartworm preventative.

11. No historical adverse drug reactions are known.

12. The dog is fed a national brand of dry dog food. It is fed two-thirds of a cup twice daily.

13. Indoor/outdoor activity (70:30) in an urban environment.

14. There are no other animals in the household.

15. The dog's appetite had been good until the current illness.

16. There has been no change in the dog's water intake.

9

17. The dog has needed to go outside to urinate more often, and she passes a large amount of urine each time. Early in the course of the problem, she also urinated inside the house one time in the middle of the night. Because the pool of urine was by the back door, the owners believe that she tried to get outside. The urine on that occasion was very pale yellow. No straining or apparent discomfort has been observed during urination, and defecation is normal.

18. The dog has lost some weight over the last 3 months.

19. The dog is slightly thin. She is alert and playful.

20. Locomotion is slow and difficult. The dog is ataxic and can walk only 30 to 40 feet (9 to 12 meters) before it slumps to the floor due to apparent weakness.

21. Rectal temperature: 101.5°F (38.6° C)

22. Pulse rate: 180 beats/min; the pulses are strong and regular.

23. Respiratory rate: 24 breaths/min

24. Pupillary light reflexes appear slow bilaterally. Palpebral reflexes and eye movements are normal.

25. The mucous membranes are pale pink and tacky. Capillary refill time is 4 seconds.

26. There is some hair in both ear canals but no discharge or hyperemia is seen.

27. No abnormalities are visualized or palpated.

28. Palpation of larynx and trachea are normal but a moist cough is easily elicited.

29. The submandibular, prescapular, and popliteal lymph nodes are palpable and of normal size. Axillary and inguinal lymph nodes are not palpable.

30. There are no palpable abnormalities associated with the thorax.

31. No abnormalities are ausculted in the thorax.

32. The abdomen is firm and moderately enlarged, and the dog resents efforts at deep palpation. Intra-abdominal structures are difficult to palpate because of the tense nature of the abdominal wall.

33. There are no visible abnormalities associated with the vulva.

34. There are no abnormalities observed or palpated on the skin or mammary glands.

35. There are no abnormalities observed or palpated in the limbs.

36. No abnormalities are detected on the anus or tail.

37. The owners first noticed the problem 1 week ago when the dog appeared to have a nose bleed that lasted about 5 minutes. The owners attributed this to trauma because the dog is very active and playful; however, another nose bleed that lasted about 10 minutes occurred yesterday. Most, if not all, of the bleeding appears to come from the right naris.

38. Because the dog is usually outdoors, the owners don't often see the dog's urination, but recently they have noticed that the dog stops frequently to urinate when on walks. Each time the dog urinates he seems to produce only a small amount of urine in relation to the time spent urinating. A few times they also think there may have been some blood in the urine.

39. To the owners' knowledge, only two episodes of epistaxis have occurred within the last week.

40. None.

41. The dog has been owned by the current owners since it was 8 weeks of age.

42. The last vaccination was given 8 months ago and included distemper virus, parainfluenza, adenovirus-2, parvovirus, coronavirus, bordetella, and rabies.

43. The dog was neutered at 18 months of age. He was hit by a car when he was 4 years old and was sucessfully treated for shock, pulmonary contusions, fractured ribs, and a fractured humerus.

44. The cat resides in northern New Mexico (southwestern United States) and has never left the area.

45. The dog had a litter of puppies when she was 3 years old, another litter when she was 4 years old, and a final litter when she was 6 years old. Estrus was last observed approximately 18 months ago.

46. The dog is not receiving any medications.

47. The dog is fed a national brand of dry dog food. It is fed 3 cups twice daily.

48. Primarily indoor activity, but with free run of a large, fenced yard when she goes outside.

49. There is another (healthy) Great Dane on the premises, which shows no signs of illness.

50. The dog's appetite remains good.

51. The dog has been drinking less since the clinical signs began.

52. Urination is normal. During the episodes of diarrhea, the feces are soft to fluid, dark brown, and occasionally contain fresh blood. Between episodes the feces appear normal.

53. The owner believes that the dog has become deaf over the last 6 months.

54. The dog is alert, active, and in good body condition.

55. The dog is slightly thin. She is alert and playful.

56. The dog is in lateral recumbency and will not/cannot rise.

57. Rectal temperature: 102.2°F (39.0°C)

58. Pulse rate: 124 beats/min; the pulses are strong and regular.

59. Respiratory rate: panting

60. Both eyes appear grossly normal. Palpebral reflexes, pupillary light reflexes (direct and consensual), and eye movements are normal.

61. Oral examination is normal except that several petechial hemorrhages are noted on the gingiva above the upper dental arcade bilaterally.

62. Otic examination is normal.

63. Palpations of larynx and trachea are normal and do not elicit a cough.

64. The submandibular, prescapular, and popliteal lymph nodes are palpable and moderately enlarged.

65. Moderate decrease in anterior chest compressibility.

66. Breath sounds are mildly increased over both lung fields.

67. The bladder is fairly small and the dog seems uncomfortable on palpation of the caudal abdomen. No other abnormalities are palpable.

68. The penis and prepuce appear normal. Rectal examination reveals a small, firm, symmetrical, nonpainful prostate gland.

69. The owner first noticed the problem 3 days ago.

70. During an episode the feces are soft to fluid, dark brown, and occasionally contain fresh blood. The first episode occurred 3 months ago and episodes have recurred every 2 to 3 weeks since then. Each episode lasts 4 to 8 days.

71. The clinical signs progressed quickly to profound weakness.

72. The dog has been owned by the current owners since it was 6 months of age.

73. The last vaccination was given 6 months ago and included distemper virus, parainfluenza, adenovirus-2, parvovirus, coronavirus, and rabies.

74. The dog has never had a prior illness.

75. The dog resides in the northeastern United States.

76. The dog was neutered at 18 months of age.

77. The cat is not receiving any medications.

78. The dog is fed a locally produced canned dog food ("Chok Full'o'Meat").

79. Indoor/outdoor activity (70:30) in a suburban environment.

80. There are no other animals on the premises.

81. The lethargy was first noticed 3 days ago and the vomiting began last night.

82. Episodes of weakness were associated with excitement (playing, chasing a cat). The dog would become weak in the hind end, then collapse to a sternal position or on its side. Recovery was rapid and the dog seemed normal within a few minutes.

83. The episodes are lasting a bit longer more recently.

84. The cat was treated successfully for a cat-fight--induced abscess on the face 14 months ago.

85. The dog resides in the southeastern United States.

86. The dog is very depressed, ataxic, and can only walk 30 to 40 feet (9 to 12 meters) before it slumps to the floor due to apparent weakness. The dog is holding its neck extended and is reluctant to move it in any direction. The dog is in thin body condition.

87. Pulse rate: 144 beats/min; the pulses are strong and regular.

88. The abdomen seems slightly distended and the dog is mildly uncomfortable on palpation. Distinct structures cannot be identified because the dog tenses her abdominal muscles.

89. The owner first noticed the problem 30 minutes ago.

90. The dog's appetite has slowly decreased during the past few days. Today she would not eat anything.

91. Water intake is unknown because the dog drinks from a large tub of water outside (various family members fill it when it is low) as well as from the other animals' water sources.

92. Urination and defecation had been normal but have decreased in amount and frequency during the last 3 days.

93. She sometimes has 1- to 2-hour periods when she is quieter and less active than normal.

94. The dog is quiet but alert. He is lean, but the owners report that he has never been a heavy dog. By referring to his record, you find that he has lost approximately 4.4 lb (2 kg) since his last visit 10 months ago.

95. The dog prefers to lie on the floor, but locomotion is normal when she is encouraged to get up and walk around.

96. Rectal temperature: 99.1° F (37.3°C)

97. Pulse rate: 170 beats/min. The pulses are weak and regular.

98. Respiratory rate: 32 breaths/min

99. The mucous membranes are pale pink and tacky. Capillary refill time is 2 to 3 seconds.

100. Ear canals are normal, but there are several petechial hemorrhages noted on the inside of both pinnae.

101. Breath sounds are moderately decreased over both lung fields.

102. Fluid-filled bowel loops are found on abdominal palpation. No other abnormalities are palpable.

103. The owner first noticed the coughing 2 months ago.

104. The owner noted that the dog was depressed 30 minutes ago, but since then the dog has become profoundly weak.

105. The problem is getting worse--five days ago the dog was only lethargic, but now the dog is recumbent.

106. The cat has been owned by the current owners since it was 8 weeks of age.

107. The last vaccination was given 1 month ago and included distemper virus, parainfluenza, adenovirus-2, parvovirus, coronavirus, bordetella, and rabies.

108. The dog has had intermittent flea bite dermatitis over the last 5 years.

109. The dog resides in northern Maine (northeastern United States) and has never left the area.

110. The dog was neutered at 1 year of age.

111. The dog is fed a premium quality dry food. It is fed two-thirds of a cup twice daily.

112. Primarily outdoor activity. The dog has free run of a farm and sleeps in his doghouse or in the barn on cold nights.

113. There is one other dog (a healthy female spayed German shepherd dog), several cats, three horses, and dairy cattle on the farm.

114. The cat ate well yesterday, but ate less than its normal amount today.

115. Water intake is unknown because all the dogs drink from two large bowls of water.

116. The dog is usually outdoors so the owners don't often see the dog's urination, but recently they have noticed that the dog stops frequently to urinate when on walks. Each time the dog urinates, he seems to produce only a small amount of urine in relation to the amount of time spent urinating. The owners also think that a few times there may have been some blood in the urine; they have not observed the dog defecating, but feces in the yard appear normal.

117. Over the last 2 months, the owners think the dog has tired more easily following vigorous exercise.

118. The dog, which is laterally recumbent and depressed, is carried into the clinic by the owners. The dog's mucous membranes are pale and the capillary refill time is prolonged.

119. The dog is laterally recumbent and is unable to rise.

120. Rectal temperature: 101.8°F (38.8°C)

121. Pulse rate: 80 beats/min; the pulses are strong and regular.

122. Respiratory rate: 36 breaths/min

123. Oral examination: mucous membrane color and capillary refill time are normal.

124. No abnormalities are ausculted in the thorax other than the slow heart rate.

125. There are no abnormalities on abdominal palpation.

126. A seizure was first observed 4 months ago. The dog was clinically normal after that but then had 2 more seizures in the last month.

127. The dog has needed to go outside to urinate more often and she passes a large amount of urine each time. Early in the course of the problem, she also urinated in the house one time. Because this occurred in the middle of the night and the pool of urine was by the back door, the owners believe that she tried to get outside. The urine that time was very pale yellow. No straining or apparent discomfort during urination has been observed.

128. The lethargy has been getting worse. The frequency of vomiting (approximately once every 3 to 4 hours) has not changed since last night.

129. The last vaccination was given 10 months ago and included feline panleukopenia, rhinotracheitis and calcivirus, and rabies.

130. The dog had an ovariohysterectomy at 6 months of age. There have been no prior illnesses.

131. The dog resides in southern California (southwestern United States), but has traveled extensively with the owners throughout North America in the past 2 years.

132. The dog had an ovariohysterectomy at 6 months of age.

133. The dog is fed a national brand of dry dog food *ad libitum* and is given occasional table scraps.

134. Primarily outdoor activity. The dog has free range of a large acreage.

135. There are three other (healthy) golden retrievers on the premises.

136. The dog's appetite has been poor since the clinical signs began.

137. There has been no change in the dog's water intake. The owner estimates it at 5 to 6 cups/day.

138. Defecation has decreased as her appetite has decreased. Urination may be increased slightly, but the owners are unsure because they think they may have been watching her more closely since she became ill.

139. None.

140. The dog is quiet but alert. She is thin.

141. Locomotion is normal.

142. Rectal temperature: 103.1°F (39.5°C)

143. Pulse rate: 96 beats/min; the pulses are strong and regular.

144. Respiratory rate: 40 breaths/min

145. A 2/6 systolic murmur is present with the point of maximal intensity over the mitral valve region. No abnormalities are heard over the lung fields.

146. The dog became lethargic 5 days ago. Three days ago the weakness was noticed. Today the dog would not or could not rise.

147. The dyspnea has been accompanied by a decrease in activity.

148. The problem seems to be slowly getting worse.

149. The last vaccination was given 9 months ago and included distemper virus, parainfluenza, adenovirus-2, parvovirus, coronavirus, and rabies.

150. The dog has been treated twice for otitis externa. She also had a flea infestation late last summer.

151. The dog resides in the midwestern United States.

152. The animal has never been bred.

153. The dog is fed a national brand of dry dog food *ad libitum.*

154. Indoor/outdoor activity (60:40) in a rural environment.

155. There is one other (healthy) poodle and a (healthy) cat in the household.

156. The dog's appetite has been unchanged—she has always "nibbled" her meals versus devouring them.

157. There has been no change in the dog's water intake. The owner estimates it at 7 to 8 cups/day.

158. Urination and defecation have been normal.

159. The dog is in lateral recumbency and will not/cannot rise. She is responsive to audio, visual, and tactile stimuli.

160. Rectal temperature: 99.5°F (37.5°C)

161. Pulse rate: 52 beats/min; the pulses are weak and regular.

162. Respiratory rate: 50 breaths/min

163. Mild hepatomegaly is detected on abdominal palpation. The bladder is moderately distended.

164. The problem first occurred 3 months ago and has recurred every 2 to 3 weeks since that time. Each episode lasts 4 to 8 days.

165. The dog became lethargic 5 days ago. Three days ago the weakness was noticed. Today the dog would not or could not rise.

166. The cough has gradually become more frequent over the last 2 months, and currently the dog has bouts of coughing 3 to 4 times a day.

167. The last vaccination was given 7 months ago and included distemper virus, parainfluenza, adenovirus-2, parvovirus, coronavirus, and rabies.

168. The dog has had several episodes of acute moist dermatitis (hot spots) during the summer months.

169. The dog resides in Minnesota (northern central United States) and has never traveled outside of this area.

170. The dog has had one litter of 3 healthy puppies 4 months ago.

171. The dog is fed a premium quality dry food. It is fed one-half cup twice daily.

172. Primarily outdoor activity in a large fenced yard.

173. There is one healthy cat in the household and no other dogs. The dog is leash walked when outside of its fenced yard and has limited contact with other animals.

174. Her appetite was normal until 3 days ago, but has progressively decreased since then.

175. There has been no change in the dog's water intake. The owner estimates it at 2 to 3 cups/day.

176. The owner first noticed the problem 1 to 2 weeks ago.

177. She is less active and prefers to just lie around. The vomitus contained digested food some of the time, and at other times was composed primarily of a yellow fluid.

178. The depression and lack of coordination have gradually worsened.

179. The dog had a flea infestation the past few summers and had "kennel cough" 2 years ago.

180. The dog resides in Prince Edward Island, Canada (eastern coast), and has never traveled outside of this area.

181. During the seizures the dog is recumbent, paddling, and non-responsive. During two of the three seizures she urinated. After the seizure she usually sleeps for several hours. One seizure occurred in the morning and the other two were in the evening.

182. Episodes of weakness occurred once last week and twice this week.

183. The cat is quiet and depressed. Moderate dyspnea is present. Respiratory effort is increased during both inspiration and expiration.

184. The owner first noticed that the dog was depressed 1 week ago, but the incoordination developed over the last 2 days.

185. The dog is alert and active. She is moderately overweight.

186. The owners feel that most of the bleeding occurred from the right naris. The dog sneezed intermittently during the episodes of bleeding.

187. The dog resides in the midwestern United States.

188. The dog is very quiet and prefers to lie on the floor.

189. Pulse rate: 90 beats/min; the pulses are strong and regular.

190. The dog had a litter of puppies when she was 2 years old, one when she was 3 years old, one when she was 4 years old, and a final litter when she was 6 years old. Estrus was last observed approximately 6 weeks ago; she was bred but did not become pregnant.

191. The cat is fed a premium quality dry food. It is fed one-half cup twice daily.

192. There is one other healthy cat in the household.

193. The dog's appetite decreases during the episodes of diarrhea. Between the episodes, the dog has a good appetite.

194. The dog shares a water bowl with another poodle and a cat, so individual water consumption is not known. However, at least one of the animals is drinking more; the owner has had to refill the bowl more often than is usual.

195. The dog is alert, active, and mildly overweight.

196. Rectal temperature: 102.4°F (39.1°C)

197. Pulse rate: 70 beats/min; the pulses are strong and regular.

198. The owner first noticed episodes of weakness 2 weeks ago. The dog has had three episodes since then.

199. The cough seems moist and the dog gags and swallows at the end of a bout of coughing.

200. The dyspnea has been gradual in onset over the last 3 days.

201. The dog was neutered at 7 months of age. An episode of acute vomiting attributed to garbage ingestion occurred 3 years ago.

202. The dog resides in western Canada but has traveled throughout North America with the owners. The most recent trip, 4 months ago, was to the southwestern United States.

203. The dog is fed a premium quality dry food. It is fed five cups twice daily.

204. There are two other dogs in the household, neither of which is showing clinical signs of illness.

205. The owner has not noticed a change in the cat's water intake

206. The problem has been largely unchanged since it was noticed.

207. The mucous membranes are pale and the capillary refill time is prolonged.

208. Her appetite has decreased over the last three days.

Section III

Parts C, D, and E
Diagnostic Tests

Hint: Create a problem list based on the abnormalities identified in the patient history and physical examination. For each problem, develop a list of differential diagnoses and select diagnostic tests that will allow you to efficiently develop a diagnosis or diagnoses. Assume that the owner does not have a specific cost limit, but that the charges must be justifiable (Note: The costs listed for diagnostic tests and procedures are approximations and can vary markedly depending on practice type and geographic region).

PART C **Directions:** Select your initial diagnostic tests and look up the corresponding number in the *Answers for Parts C, D, and E (Diagnostic Tests).* After you have obtained the results from your initial diagnostic tests, proceed to Part D.

PART D **Directions:** Select any further diagnostic tests and look up the corresponding number in the *Answers for Parts C, D, and E (Diagnostic Tests).* After you have obtained the results from Part D, you may make a diagnosis or diagnoses in Part F, or go to Part E and select further diagnostic tests.

PART E **Directions:** Select your final diagnostic tests and look up the corresponding number in the *Answers for Parts C, D, and E (Diagnostic Tests).* This is the last time you may select diagnostic tests. After you have obtained your final results, proceed to Part F and make a diagnosis or diagnoses.

To avoid bias and to make the case management exercise as realistic as possible, please read only the selected numbered answer.

BIOCHEMICAL TESTS

Ammonia (resting): **$18.00**

Case 1=86	Case 2=86	Case 3=86	Case 4=86	Case 5=86	Case 6=86
Case 7=86	Case 8=86	Case 9=86	Case 10=86	Case 11=179	Case 12=86

Ammonia tolerance test/ammonia challenge: **$36.00**

Case 1=87	Case 2=87	Case 3=87	Case 4=87	Case 5=87	Case 6=87
Case 7=87	Case 8=87	Case 9=87	Case 10=87	Case 11=180	Case 12=87

Arterial blood gas: $20.00

Case 1=2	Case 2=107	Case 3=2	Case 4=199	Case 5=2	Case 6=2
Case 7=2	Case 8=2	Case 9=2	Case 10=255	Case 11=2	Case 12=2

Bile acid concentrations (fasting and postprandial): $34.00

Case 1=3	Case 2=3	Case 3=3	Case 4=3	Case 5=3	Case 6=3
Case 7=3	Case 8=3	Case 9=3	Case 10=3	Case 11=108	Case 12=3

Biochemical profile: $50.00

Case 1=38	Case 2=138	Case 3=224	Case 4=272	Case 5=293	Case 6=306
Case 7=321	Case 8=306	Case 9=314	Case 10=181	Case 11=325	Case 12=186

N-benzoyl-L-tyrosyl-para-aminobenzoic acid (BT-PABA) digestion test: $130.00

Case 1=81	Case 2=81	Case 3=81	Case 4=81	Case 5=81	Case 6=81
Case 7=81	Case 8=81	Case 9=175	Case 10=81	Case 11=81	Case 12=81

Cobalamin concentration: $15.00

Case 1=78	Case 2=78	Case 3=78	Case 4=78	Case 5=78	Case 6=78
Case 7=78	Case 8=78	Case 9=172	Case 10=245	Case 11=245	Case 12=245

Folate concentration: $15.00

Case 1=79	Case 2=79	Case 3=79	Case 4=79	Case 5=79	Case 6=79
Case 7=79	Case 8=79	Case 9=173	Case 10=246	Case 11=246	Case 12=246

Osmolality (serum): $8.00

Case 1=88	Case 2=88	Case 3=88	Case 4=88	Case 5=88	Case 6=88
Case 7=88	Case 8=88	Case 9=88	Case 10=190	Case 11=88	Case 12=248

Protein electrophoresis (serum): $20.00

Case 1=89	Case 2=89	Case 3=89	Case 4=89	Case 5=89	Case 6=89
Case 7=89	Case 8=89	Case 9=89	Case 10=89	Case 11=89	Case 12=89

Trypsin-like immunoreactivity (serum): $30.00

Case 1=59	Case 2=59	Case 3=59	Case 4=155	Case 5=59	Case 6=59
Case 7=59	Case 8=59	Case 9=59	Case 10=59	Case 11=59	Case 12=59

Urine para-aminobenzoic acid (PABA) excretion test (6-hour): $50.00

Case 1=82	Case 2=82	Case 3=82	Case 4=82	Case 5=82	Case 6=82
Case 7=82	Case 8=82	Case 9=176	Case 10=82	Case 11=82	Case 12=82

Xylose absorption test: $130.00

Case 1=83	Case 2=83	Case 3=83	Case 4=83	Case 5=83	Case 6=83
Case 7=83	Case 8=83	Case 9=177	Case 10=83	Case 11=83	Case 12=83

COAGULATION TESTS

Fibrin degradation products (FDP): $23.00

Case 1=49	Case 2=49	Case 3=49	Case 4=49	Case 5=49	Case 6=49
Case 7=49	Case 8=49	Case 9=49	Case 10=49	Case 11=49	Case 12=49

Mucosal bleeding time: $18.00

Case 1=48	Case 2=48	Case 3=147	Case 4=231	Case 5=48	Case 6=48
Case 7=48	Case 8=48	Case 9=48	Case 10=48	Case 11=48	Case 12=48

Partial thromboplastin time (PTT): $15.00

Case 1=47	Case 2=47	Case 3=47	Case 4=146	Case 5=47	Case 6=47
Case 7=47	Case 8=47	Case 9=47	Case 10=47	Case 11=47	Case 12=47

Prothrombin time (PT): $15.00

Case 1=46	Case 2=46	Case 3=46	Case 4=145	Case 5=46	Case 6=46
Case 7=46	Case 8=46	Case 9=46	Case 10=46	Case 11=46	Case 12=46

von Willebrand's factor antigen: **$35.00**

Case 1=50	Case 2=50	Case 3=50	Case 4=50	Case 5=50	Case 6=50
Case 7=50	Case 8=50	Case 9=50	Case 10=50	Case 11=50	Case 12=50

ELECTRODIAGNOSTIC TESTS

Electrocardiogram: **$30.00**

Case 1=16	Case 2=121	Case 3=121	Case 4=121	Case 5=121	Case 6=121
Case 7=121	Case 8=121	Case 9=121	Case 10=210	Case 11=121	Case 12=121

Electromyogram: **$80.00**

Case 1=17	Case 2=17	Case 3=17	Case 4=122	Case 5=17	Case 6=17
Case 7=17	Case 8=17	Case 9=17	Case 10=122	Case 11=17	Case 12=17

Nerve conduction studies: **$80.00**

Case 1=26	Case 2=26	Case 3=26	Case 4=129	Case 5=26	Case 6=26
Case 7=26	Case 8=26	Case 9=26	Case 10=129	Case 11=215	Case 12=26

ENDOCRINOLOGIC TESTS

Adrenocorticotropic hormone (ACTH) concentration (endogenous): **$70.00**

Case 1=91	Case 2=91	Case 3=91	Case 4=326	Case 5=91	Case 6=91
Case 7=91	Case 8=91	Case 9=91	Case 10=191	Case 11=91	Case 12=91

Adrenocorticotropic hormone (ACTH) stimulation test: **$40.00**

Case 1=1	Case 2=1	Case 3=1	Case 4=1	Case 5=1	Case 6=1
Case 7=106	Case 8=1	Case 9=1	Case 10=198	Case 11=1	Case 12=1

Cannot be done the same day as low-dose or high-dose dexamethasone suppression test.

Dexamethasone suppression test (low-dose): **$50.00**

Case 1=21	Case 2=21	Case 3=21	Case 4=21	Case 5=21	Case 6=21
Case 7=124	Case 8=21	Case 9=21	Case 10=211	Case 11=21	Case 12=21

Cannot be done the same day as the adrenocorticotropic hormone (ACTH) stimulation test or the high-dose dexamethasone suppression test.

Dexamethasone suppression test (high-dose): $50.00

Case 1=22	Case 2=22	Case 3=22	Case 4=22	Case 5=22	Case 6=22
Case 7=125	Case 8=22	Case 9=22	Case 10=212	Case 11=22	Case 12=22

Cannot be done the same day as the adrenocorticotropic hormone (ACTH) stimulation test or the low-dose dexamethasone suppression test.

Glucose tolerance test: $50.00

Case 1=23	Case 2=23	Case 3=23	Case 4=23	Case 5=23	Case 6=23
Case 7=126	Case 8=23	Case 9=23	Case 10=23	Case 11=23	Case 12=23

Insulin concentration (fasting, endogenous): $40.00

Case 1=18	Case 2=18	Case 3=18	Case 4=18	Case 5=18	Case 6=18
Case 7=123	Case 8=18	Case 9=18	Case 10=18	Case 11=18	Case 12=18

Parathyroid hormone (PTH) concentration: $50.00

Case 1=92	Case 2=92	Case 3=92	Case 4=92	Case 5=92	Case 6=92
Case 7=92	Case 8=92	Case 9=92	Case 10=92	Case 11=92	Case 12=92

Thyroid stimulating hormone (TSH) concentration (endogenous): $25.00

Case 1=93	Case 2=93	Case 3=93	Case 4=93	Case 5=93	Case 6=93
Case 7=93	Case 8=93	Case 9=93	Case 10=93	Case 11=93	Case 12=93

Thyroxine (T₄) concentration (resting endogenous): $15.00

Case 1=35	Case 2=137	Case 3=35	Case 4=223	Case 5=35	Case 6=137
Case 7=271	Case 8=35	Case 9=271	Case 10=271	Case 11=271	Case 12=271

Urine cortisol:creatinine ratio: $25.00

Case 1=94	Case 2=94	Case 3=94	Case 4=94	Case 5=94	Case 6=94
Case 7=192	Case 8=94	Case 9=94	Case 10=249	Case 11=94	Case 12=94

Water deprivation/vasopressin response test: $100.00

Case 1=24	Case 2=127	Case 3=24	Case 4=24	Case 5=213	Case 6=24
Case 7=262	Case 8=24	Case 9=24	Case 10=291	Case 11=304	Case 12=313

ENDOSCOPY

Bronchoscopy—examination and sampling: $150.00

Case 1=95	Case 2=95	Case 3=193	Case 4=95	Case 5=250	Case 6=193
Case 7=193	Case 8=193	Case 9=193	Case 10=95	Case 11=287	Case 12=300

Colonoscopy and proctoscopy—examination and biopsy: $150.00

Case 1=55	Case 2=151	Case 3=151	Case 4=55	Case 5=151	Case 6=151
Case 7=151	Case 8=151	Case 9=234	Case 10=55	Case 11=151	Case 12=151

Gastroduodenoscopy—examination and biopsy: $150.00

Case 1=54	Case 2=150	Case 3=150	Case 4=54	Case 5=150	Case 6=150
Case 7=150	Case 8=150	Case 9=233	Case 10=54	Case 11=278	Case 12=330

Rhinoscopy—examination and biopsy: $150.00

Case 1=73	Case 2=73	Case 3=168	Case 4=73	Case 5=242	Case 6=242
Case 7=242	Case 8=242	Case 9=242	Case 10=73	Case 11=284	Case 12=242

HEMATOLOGY

Complete blood count: $20.00

Case 1=7	Case 2=112	Case 3=202	Case 4=37	Case 5=289	Case 6=302
Case 7=311	Case 8=311	Case 9=319	Case 10=324	Case 11=311	Case 12=184

IMMUNOLOGICAL TESTS

Acetylcholine receptor antibody titer (serum): $40.00

Case 1=36	Case 2=36	Case 3=36	Case 4=36	Case 5=36	Case 6=36
Case 7=36	Case 8=36	Case 9=36	Case 10=36	Case 11=36	Case 12=36

Coomb's test: **$20.00**

Case 1=90	Case 2=90	Case 3=90	Case 4=90	Case 5=90	Case 6=90
Case 7=90	Case 8=90	Case 9=90	Case 10=90	Case 11=90	Case 12=90

MEDICAL PROCEDURES

Abdominocentesis and fluid analysis: **$30.00**

Case 1=44	Case 2=143	Case 3=44	Case 4=44	Case 5=44	Case 6=44
Case 7=44	Case 8=44	Case 9=44	Case 10=44	Case 11=44	Case 12=229

Aspirate—lymph node: **$20.00**

Case 1=58	Case 2=58	Case 3=58	Case 4=58	Case 5=58	Case 6=154
Case 7=58	Case 8=58	Case 9=58	Case 10=58	Case 11=58	Case 12=58

Aspirate—mass: **$20.00**

Case 1=76	Case 2=244	Case 3=76	Case 4=171	Case 5=76	Case 6=76
Case 7=76	Case 8=286	Case 9=76	Case 10=76	Case 11=76	Case 12=76

Biopsy—liver: **$100.00**

Case 1=61	Case 2=61	Case 3=157	Case 4=237	Case 5=61	Case 6=61
Case 7=281	Case 8=61	Case 9=61	Case 10=237	Case 11=299	Case 12=61

Biopsy—muscle: **$180.00**

Case 1=25	Case 2=25	Case 3=128	Case 4=214	Case 5=25	Case 6=25
Case 7=25	Case 8=25	Case 9=25	Case 10=214	Case 11=263	Case 12=25

Biopsy—peripheral nerve: **$180.00**

Case 1=28	Case 2=28	Case 3=131	Case 4=217	Case 5=28	Case 6=28
Case 7=28	Case 8=28	Case 9=28	Case 10=217	Case 11=265	Case 12=28

Bone marrow aspirate and cytologic evaluation: $60.00

Case 1=57	Case 2=57	Case 3=153	Case 4=57	Case 5=57	Case 6=57
Case 7=57	Case 8=57	Case 9=57	Case 10=57	Case 11=57	Case 12=57

Cardiac catheterization: $300.00

Case 1=5	Case 2=110	Case 3=200	Case 4=5	Case 5=200	Case 6=200
Case 7=200	Case 8=200	Case 9=200	Case 10=256	Case 11=328	Case 12=200

Cerebrospinal fluid (CSF) collection and analysis: $100.00

Case 1=6	Case 2=6	Case 3=6	Case 4=111	Case 5=6	Case 6=201
Case 7=6	Case 8=6	Case 9=257	Case 10=111	Case 11=6	Case 12=6

Fat absorption test: $25.00

Case 1=80	Case 2=80	Case 3=80	Case 4=80	Case 5=80	Case 6=80
Case 7=80	Case 8=80	Case 9=174	Case 10=247	Case 11=80	Case 12=247

Fundoscopic examination: $20.00

Case 1=63	Case 2=63	Case 3=159	Case 4=63	Case 5=63	Case 6=239
Case 7=63	Case 8=63	Case 9=63	Case 10=63	Case 11=63	Case 12=63

Nasal flush (traumatic): $150.00

Case 1=74	Case 2=74	Case 3=169	Case 4=74	Case 5=243	Case 6=243
Case 7=243	Case 8=243	Case 9=243	Case 10=74	Case 11=285	Case 12=243

Neurologic examination: $30.00

Case 1=27	Case 2=130	Case 3=27	Case 4=27	Case 5=27	Case 6=216
Case 7=27	Case 8=27	Case 9=27	Case 10=264	Case 11=27	Case 12=27

Pericardiocentesis: $50.00

Case 1=105	Case 2=105	Case 3=197	Case 4=105	Case 5=105	Case 6=105
Case 7=105	Case 8=105	Case 9=105	Case 10=254	Case 11=105	Case 12=105

Rectal scraping cytology: $20.00

Case 1=96	Case 2=96	Case 3=96	Case 4=96	Case 5=96	Case 6=96
Case 7=96	Case 8=96	Case 9=96	Case 10=96	Case 11=96	Case 12=96

Tensilon (edrophonium chloride) response test: $25.00

Case 1=39	Case 2=39	Case 3=39	Case 4=39	Case 5=39	Case 6=39
Case 7=39	Case 8=39	Case 9=39	Case 10=39	Case 11=39	Case 12=39

Thoracocentesis and fluid analysis and culture: $30.00

Case 1=75	Case 2=75	Case 3=75	Case 4=170	Case 5=75	Case 6=75
Case 7=75	Case 8=75	Case 9=75	Case 10=75	Case 11=75	Case 12=75

Transtracheal wash and fluid analysis and culture: $70.00

Case 1=53	Case 2=53	Case 3=149	Case 4=232	Case 5=277	Case 6=53
Case 7=53	Case 8=53	Case 9=53	Case 10=298	Case 11=53	Case 12=53

MICROBIOLOGY

Duodenal aspirate culture (quantitative): $150.00

Case 1=85	Case 2=178	Case 3=85	Case 4=178	Case 5=85	Case 6=85
Case 7=85	Case 8=85	Case 9=85	Case 10=178	Case 11=329	Case 12=85

Fecal culture: $25.00

Case 1=84	Case 2=84	Case 3=84	Case 4=84	Case 5=84	Case 6=84
Case 7=84	Case 8=84	Case 9=84	Case 10=84	Case 11=84	Case 12=84

Urine culture: $25.00

Case 1=43	Case 2=43	Case 3=142	Case 4=43	Case 5=43	Case 6=43
Case 7=228	Case 8=43	Case 9=43	Case 10=43	Case 11=43	Case 12=43

PARASITOLOGY

Baermann fecal flotation: $20.00

Case 1=52	Case 2=52	Case 3=52	Case 4=52	Case 5=148	Case 6=52
Case 7=52	Case 8=52	Case 9=52	Case 10=52	Case 11=52	Case 12=52

Fecal flotation and direct examination—routine: $15.00

Case 1=51	Case 2=51	Case 3=51	Case 4=51	Case 5=51	Case 6=51
Case 7=51	Case 8=51	Case 9=51	Case 10=51	Case 11=51	Case 12=51

Heartworm antigen test: $20.00

Case 1=19	Case 2=19	Case 3=19	Case 4=19	Case 5=19	Case 6=19
Case 7=19	Case 8=19	Case 9=19	Case 10=19	Case 11=19	Case 12=19

Heartworm microfilaria recovery test (e.g., modified Knott's test): $15.00

Case 1=20	Case 2=20	Case 3=20	Case 4=20	Case 5=20	Case 6=20
Case 7=20	Case 8=20	Case 9=20	Case 10=20	Case 11=20	Case 12=20

RADIOLOGY

Computerized tomography—abdomen: $300.00

Case 1=9	Case 2=114	Case 3=9	Case 4=9	Case 5=9	Case 6=9
Case 7=204	Case 8=258	Case 9=290	Case 10=303	Case 11=312	Case 12=320

Computerized tomography—skull: $300.00

Case 1=8	Case 2=8	Case 3=8	Case 4=113	Case 5=8	Case 6=8
Case 7=8	Case 8=8	Case 9=8	Case 10=113	Case 11=203	Case 12=8

Contrast radiographs—cystogram: $85.00

Case 1=13	Case 2=13	Case 3=13	Case 4=13	Case 5=13	Case 6=13
Case 7=13	Case 8=118	Case 9=13	Case 10=208	Case 11=260	Case 12=331

Contrast radiographs—diskogram (lumbosacral): $110.00

Case 1=11	Case 2=11	Case 3=11	Case 4=116	Case 5=11	Case 6=11
Case 7=11	Case 8=11	Case 9=11	Case 10=116	Case 11=206	Case 12=11

Contrast radiographs—epidurogram: $150.00

Case 1=12	Case 2=12	Case 3=12	Case 4=117	Case 5=12	Case 6=12
Case 7=12	Case 8=12	Case 9=12	Case 10=117	Case 11=207	Case 12=12

Contrast radiographs—intravenous pyelogram (IVP): $110.00

Case 1=15	Case 2=15	Case 3=15	Case 4=15	Case 5=15	Case 6=15
Case 7=15	Case 8=15	Case 9=15	Case 10=120	Case 11=15	Case 12=332

Contrast radiographs—myelogram: $200.00

Case 1=10	Case 2=10	Case 3=10	Case 4=115	Case 5=10	Case 6=205
Case 7=10	Case 8=10	Case 9=10	Case 10=115	Case 11=259	Case 12=10

Contrast radiographs—splenoportogram: $250.00

Case 1=60	Case 2=156	Case 3=236	Case 4=60	Case 5=156	Case 6=156
Case 7=156	Case 8=156	Case 9=156	Case 10=60	Case 11=280	Case 12=333

Contrast radiographs—upper gastrointestinal study: $110.00

Case 1=14	Case 2=14	Case 3=14	Case 4=14	Case 5=14	Case 6=14
Case 7=14	Case 8=14	Case 9=119	Case 10=209	Case 11=14	Case 12=334

Fluoroscopy—gastric: $80.00

Case 1=98	Case 2=98	Case 3=98	Case 4=98	Case 5=98	Case 6=98
Case 7=98	Case 8=98	Case 9=98	Case 10=195	Case 11=98	Case 12=252

Fluoroscopy—thorax: $80.00

Case 1=97	Case 2=97	Case 3=97	Case 4=194	Case 5=97	Case 6=97
Case 7=97	Case 8=97	Case 9=97	Case 10=251	Case 11=97	Case 12=97

Survey radiographs—abdominal: $50.00

Case 1=30	Case 2=133	Case 3=30	Case 4=30	Case 5=30	Case 6=30
Case 7=219	Case 8=30	Case 9=267	Case 10=30	Case 11=292	Case 12=305

Survey radiographs (with anesthesia)—cervical spine: $95.00

Case 1=31	Case 2=31	Case 3=31	Case 4=31	Case 5=31	Case 6=134
Case 7=31	Case 8=31	Case 9=31	Case 10=220	Case 11=268	Case 12=31

Survey radiographs (with anesthesia)—lumbosacral spine: **$95.00**

Case 1=33	Case 2=33	Case 3=33	Case 4=33	Case 5=33	Case 6=136
Case 7=33	Case 8=33	Case 9=33	Case 10=222	Case 11=270	Case 12=33

Survey radiographs (with anesthesia)—nasal series: **$125.00**

Case 1=72	Case 2=72	Case 3=167	Case 4=72	Case 5=241	Case 6=241
Case 7=241	Case 8=241	Case 9=241	Case 10=72	Case 11=283	Case 12=241

Survey radiographs (with anesthesia)—thoracolumbar spine: **$95.00**

Case 1=32	Case 2=32	Case 3=32	Case 4=32	Case 5=32	Case 6=135
Case 7=32	Case 8=32	Case 9=32	Case 10=221	Case 11=269	Case 12=32

Survey radiographs—thorax: **$50.00**

Case 1=29	Case 2=132	Case 3=132	Case 4=218	Case 5=266	Case 6=132
Case 7=132	Case 8=132	Case 9=132	Case 10=188	Case 11=132	Case 12=132

Survey radiographs—pelvis/hips: **$50.00**

Case 1=34	Case 2=34	Case 3=34	Case 4=34	Case 5=34	Case 6=34
Case 7=34	Case 8=34	Case 9=34	Case 10=34	Case 11=34	Case 12=34

Ultrasound—cardiac: **$95.00**

Case 1=40	Case 2=139	Case 3=225	Case 4=273	Case 5=225	Case 6=225
Case 7=225	Case 8=225	Case 9=225	Case 10=294	Case 11=225	Case 12=225

Ultrasound—abdomen: **$80.00**

Case 1=41	Case 2=140	Case 3=41	Case 4=41	Case 5=41	Case 6=41
Case 7=226	Case 8=274	Case 9=295	Case 10=41	Case 11=307	Case 12=315

SEROLOGIC TESTS

Aspergillus serology: **$30.00**

Case 1=70	Case 2=70	Case 3=70	Case 4=70	Case 5=70	Case 6=70
Case 7=70	Case 8=70	Case 9=70	Case 10=70	Case 11=70	Case 12=70

Cryptococcal capsular antigen test: $30.00

Case 1=69	Case 2=69	Case 3=69	Case 4=69	Case 5=69	Case 6=165
Case 7=69	Case 8=69	Case 9=69	Case 10=69	Case 11=69	Case 12=69

Ehrlichia canis *titer:* $30.00

Case 1=67	Case 2=67	Case 3=67	Case 4=163	Case 5=67	Case 6=67
Case 7=67	Case 8=67	Case 9=67	Case 10=67	Case 11=67	Case 12=67

Rocky Mountain spotted fever (Ricksettsia rickettsii) *titer:* $30.00

Case 1=68	Case 2=68	Case 3=68	Case 4=164	Case 5=240	Case 6=68
Case 7=240	Case 8=240	Case 9=240	Case 10=240	Case 11=240	Case 12=240

Toxoplasma gondii *(serum IgG and IgM) titer:* $30.00

Case 1=71	Case 2=71	Case 3=71	Case 4=166	Case 5=71	Case 6=71
Case 7=71	Case 8=71	Case 9=71	Case 10=71	Case 11=71	Case 12=71

SURGICAL PROCEDURES

Laparotomy (exploratory): $250.00

Case 1=45	Case 2=144	Case 3=230	Case 4=45	Case 5=276	Case 6=276
Case 7=297	Case 8=309	Case 9=317	Case 10=45	Case 11=323	Case 12=183

Laparotomy and intestinal biopsy: $400.00

Case 1=56	Case 2=152	Case 3=235	Case 4=56	Case 5=152	Case 6=152
Case 7=152	Case 8=152	Case 9=279	Case 10=56	Case 11=152	Case 12=335

Rhinotomy: $450.00

Case 1=62	Case 2=158	Case 3=238	Case 4=62	Case 5=158	Case 6=158
Case 7=158	Case 8=158	Case 9=158	Case 10=62	Case 11=282	Case 12=158

Thoracotomy: $700.00

Case 1=99	Case 2=99	Case 3=196	Case 4=253	Case 5=288	Case 6=301
Case 7=318	Case 8=318	Case 9=318	Case 10=99	Case 11=318	Case 12=318

URINE TESTS

Endogenous creatinine clearance: $50.00

Case 1=4	Case 2=4	Case 3=4	Case 4=109	Case 5=4	Case 6=4
Case 7=4	Case 8=4	Case 9=4	Case 10=4	Case 11=4	Case 12=4

Urinalysis: $15.00

Case 1=42	Case 2=42	Case 3=141	Case 4=227	Case 5=275	Case 6=296
Case 7=308	Case 8=316	Case 9=322	Case 10=182	Case 11=185	Case 12=187

Urine protein:creatinine ratio: $20.00

Case 1=100	Case 2=100	Case 3=100	Case 4=100	Case 5=100	Case 6=100
Case 7=100	Case 8=327	Case 9=100	Case 10=100	Case 11=100	Case 12=100

VIRAL TESTS

Coronavirus (electron microscopy)—feces: $40.00

Case 1=102	Case 2=102	Case 3=102	Case 4=102	Case 5=102	Case 6=102
Case 7=102	Case 8=102	Case 9=102	Case 10=102	Case 11=102	Case 12=102

Distemper (cytology—conjunctival scraping): $20.00

Case 1=101	Case 2=101	Case 3=101	Case 4=189	Case 5=101	Case 6=101
Case 7=101	Case 8=101	Case 9=101	Case 10=101	Case 11=101	Case 12=101

Feline immunodeficiency virus test—enzyme-linked immunosorbent assay (ELISA): $20.00

Case 1=65	Case 2=65	Case 3=65	Case 4=161	Case 5=65	Case 6=65
Case 7=65	Case 8=65	Case 9=65	Case 10=65	Case 11=65	Case 12=65

Feline infectious peritonitis virus titer: *$30.00*

Case 1=66	Case 2=66	Case 3=66	Case 4=162	Case 5=66	Case 6=66
Case 7=66	Case 8=66	Case 9=66	Case 10=66	Case 11=66	Case 12=66

Feline leukemia virus—enzyme-linked immunosorbent assay (ELISA): *$20.00*

Case 1=64	Case 2=64	Case 3=64	Case 4=160	Case 5=64	Case 6=64
Case 7=64	Case 8=64	Case 9=64	Case 10=64	Case 11=64	Case 12=64

Parvovirus (electron microscopy—feces): *$40.00*

Case 1=103	Case 2=103	Case 3=103	Case 4=103	Case 5=103	Case 6=103
Case 7=103	Case 8=103	Case 9=103	Case 10=103	Case 11=103	Case 12=103

Parvovirus (enzyme-linked immunosorbent assay [ELISA]—feces): *$20.00*

Case 1=104	Case 2=104	Case 3=104	Case 4=104	Case 5=104	Case 6=104
Case 7=104	Case 8=104	Case 9=104	Case 10=104	Case 11=104	Case 12=104

Answers for Parts C, D, and E
(Diagnostic Tests)

1. Adrenocorticotropic Hormone (ACTH) Stimulation Test

Parameter	Result	Normal Values (dogs)	Normal Values (cats)
Baseline cortisol	98 nmol/L (3.6 μg/dl)	25–125 nmol/L (0.91–4.5 μg/dl)	15–150 nmol/L (0.54–5.4 μg/dl)
Post-ACTH cortisol	410 nmol/L (14.9 μg/dl)	200–550 nmol/L (7.2–20 μg/dl)	130–450 nmol/L (4.7–16.3 μg/dl)

2. Arterial Blood Gas Analysis

Parameter	Result	Normal Values
pH	7.39	7.351–7.463
PCO_2	36 mmHg	30.8–42.8 mmHg
PO_2	94 mmHg	80.9–103.3 mmHg
HCO_3^-	21.1 mEq/L (mmol/L)	18.8–25.6 mEq/L

HCO_3^- = bicarbonate; PCO_2 = partial pressure of carbon dioxide; pH = –log hydrogen ion concentration; PO_2 = partial pressure of oxygen.

3. Bile Acid Concentrations

Parameter	Result	Normal Values
Fasting	3.2 mg/L (8 μmol/L)	<4 mg/L (<10 μmol/L)
Postprandial	4.8 mg/L (12 μmol/L)	<8 mg/L (<20 μmol/L)

4. Endogenous creatinine clearance: 3.4 ml/min/kg (normal = 3.7 ± 0.8)

5. Cardiac catheterization: As catheters are being placed in the heart, ventricular tachycardia develops, which progresses to fibrillation and arrest. Cardiopulmonary resuscitation is unsuccessful.

6. Cerebrospinal Fluid Collection and Analysis

Parameter	Result	Normal Values
Protein	0.15 g/L (15 mg/dl)	0.10–0.30 g/L (10–30 mg/dl)
Nucleated cells	0.002 × 10⁹/L	0.0–0.002 × 10⁹/L

Cells are composed primarily of small mononuclear cells.
There are no clinical indications in this patient warranting such an invasive diagnostic procedure.

7. Complete Blood Count

Parameter	Traditional Units	SI Units	Normal Values Traditional Units	Normal Values SI Units
Hemoglobin	16 g/dl	160 g/L	13.2–19.2 g/dl	132–193 g/L
Hematocrit	51.4%	0.514 L/L	38–57%	0.38–0.57 L/L
Erythrocytes	7.28 × 10⁶/μl	7.28 × 10¹²/L	5.6–8.5 × 10⁶/μl	5.6–8.5 × 10¹²/L
MCV	70.6 mm³	70.6 fl	62–71 mm³	62–71 fl
MCH	25 pg	25 pg	22–25 pg	22–25 pg
MCHC	35.4%	354 g/L	33.7–36.5%	337–365 g/L
Reticulocytes	0%	0%	0–1.5%	0–1.5%
Platelets	401 × 10³/μl	401 × 10⁹/L	145–440 × 10³/μl	145–440 × 10⁹/L
Total nucleated cell count	8.8 × 10³/μl	8.8 × 10⁹/L	6.1–17.4 × 10³/μl	6.1–17.4 × 10⁹/L
Neutrophils	7.2 × 10³/μl (82%)	7.2 × 10⁹/L (82%)	3.9–12 × 10³/μl	3.9–12 × 10⁹/L
Band neutrophils	0	0	0–1.0 × 10³/μl	0–1.0 × 10⁹/L
Lymphocytes	0.79 × 10³/μl (9%)	0.79 × 10⁹/L (9%)	0.8–3.6 × 10³/μl	0.8–3.6 × 10⁹/L
Monocytes	0.70 × 10³/μl (8%)	0.70 × 10⁹/L (8%)	0–1.8 × 10³/μl	0–1.8 × 10⁹/L
Eosinophils	0.09 × 10³/μl (1%)	0.09 × 10⁹/L (1%)	0–1.9 × 10³/μl	0–1.9 × 10⁹/L
Basophils	0	0	0–0.2 × 10³/μl	0–0.2 × 10⁹/L

MCH = mean corpuscular hemoglobin; MCHC = mean corpuscular hemoglobin concentration; MCV = mean corpuscular volume.

8. Computerized tomography—skull: normal

9. Computerized tomography—abdomen: no abnormal findings

10. Contrast radiographs—myelogram: Normal. There are no clinical indications warranting such an invasive diagnostic procedure on this animal.

11. Contrast radiographs—diskogram (lumbosacral): Normal. There are no clinical indications warranting such as invasive diagnostic procedure in this animal.

12. Contrast radiographs—epidurogram: Normal. There are no clinical indications warranting such an invasive diagnostic procedure in this animal.

13. Contrast radiographs—cystogram: no abnormal findings

14. Contrast radiographs—upper gastrointestinal (GI): no abnormal findings

15. Contrast radiographs—intravenous pyelogram: No abnormal findings. Although the risks associated with intravenous contrast administration are low, they are present. In this case the evidence of abnormalities is insufficient to warrant this procedure. If available, ultrasound would be a safer and less invasive way to visualize the kidneys.

16. Electrocardiogram: Frequent ventricular premature contractions; approximately 25/min. A paroxysm of ventricular tachycardia occurs lasting 2 seconds.

17. Electromyography: no abnormalities identified

18. Fasting serum insulin concentration: 89 pmol/L [12.4 μU/ml] (normal: 35—200 pmol/L [4.9—27.9 μU/ml])

19. Heartworm antigen test: negative

20. Heartworm microfilaria recovery test (e.g., modified Knott test): negative

21. **Low-Dose Dexamethasone Response Test**

Parameter	Result	Normal Values (dogs)	Normal Values (cats)
Baseline cortisol	102 nmol/L (3.7 μg/dl)	25–125 nmol/L (0.91–4.5 μg/dl)	15–150 nmol/L (0.54–5.4 μg/dl)
4–hour cortisol	35 nmol/L (1.2 μg/dl)		
8–hour cortisol	26 nmol/L (0.9 μg/dl)	< 40 nmol/L (< 1.4 μg/dl)	< 40 nmol/L (< 1.4 μg/dl)

22. **High-Dose Dexamethasone Response Test**

Parameter	Result	Normal Values (dogs)	Normal Values (cats)
Baseline cortisol	89 nmol/L (3.3 μg/dl)	25–125 nmol/L (0.91–4.5 μg/dl)	15–150 nmol/L (0.54–5.4 μg/dl)
4–hour cortisol	12 nmol/L (0.4 μg/dl)		
8–hour cortisol	9 nmol/L (0.3 μg/dl)	< 50% of baseline = pituitary dependent hyperadrenocorticism in a dog with known hyperadrenocorticism	< 40 nmol/L (< 1.4 μg/dl)

23. Glucose tolerance test: normal. There are no clinical signs or test results warranting this procedure in this patient.

24. Water deprivation/vasopressin response test: Urine specific gravity is already ≥ 1.035, so there is no need for the test.

25. Muscle biopsy: left cranial tibialis muscle—no abnormal findings. There are no clinical signs or test results warranting such an invasive diagnostic procedure in this animal.

26. Nerve conduction studies: Conduction velocity normal in all peripheral nerves tested. There are no clinical signs or test results warranting this procedure in this animal.

27. Neurologic examination: no abnormal findings

28. Peripheral nerve biopsy—right distal peroneal nerve: No abnormal findings. There are no clinical indications warranting such an invasive diagnostic test in this animal.

29. Survey radiographs—thoracic: mild generalized cardiomegaly and mild left atrial enlargement. No abnormalities detected in the lung fields or pulmonary vasculatase.

30. Survey radiographs—abdominal: no abnormal findings

31. Survey radiographs—cervical spine: No abnormal findings. There are no clinical signs or test results warranting this procedure (which requires general anesthesia) in this patient.

32. Survey radiographs—thoracolumbar spine: No abnormal findings. There are no clinical signs or test results warranting this procedure (which requires general anesthesia) in this patient.

33. Survey radiographs—lumbosacral spine: No abnormal findings. There are no clinical signs or test results warranting this procedure (which requires general anesthesia) in this patient.

34. Survey radiographs—hips/pelvis: no abnormal findings

35. Baseline serum T_4 (thyroxine) concentration: 22 nmol/L [1.7 μg/dl] (normal values: 12–50 nmol/L [0.9–3.9 μg/dl])

36. Serum acetylcholine receptor antibody: 0.2 nmol/L (normal value: < 0.6 nmol/L)

37. Complete Blood Count

Parameter	Traditional Units	SI Units	Normal Values Traditional Units	Normal Values SI Units
Hemoglobin	15.0 g/dl	150 g/L	8.0–15.0 g/dl	80–150 g/L
Hematocrit	45%	0.45 L/L	24–45%	0.24–0.45 L/L
Erythrocytes	$10.0 \times 10^6/\mu l$	$10.0 \times 10^{12}/L$	$5.0–10 \times 10^6/\mu l$	$5.0–10 \times 10^{12}/L$
MCV	45.9 mm^3	45.9 fl	39–50 mm^3	39–50 fl
MCH	15 pg	15 pg	13–17 pg	13–17 pg
MCHC	32.6%	326 g/L	32–36%	320–360 g/L
Reticulocytes	0%	0%	0–1.5%	0–1.5%
Platelets	$210 \times 10^3/\mu l$	$210 \times 10^9/L$	$190–400 \times 10^3/\mu l$	$190–400 \times 10^9/L$
Total nucleated cell count	$9.4 \times 10^3/\mu l$	$9.4 \times 10^9/L$	$5.5–15.4 \times 10^3/\mu l$	$5.5–15.4 \times 10^9/L$
Neutrophils	$8.0 \times 10^3/\mu l$ (85%)	$8.0 \times 10^9/L$ (85%)	$2.5–12.5 \times 10^3/\mu l$	$2.5–12.5 \times 10^9/L$
Band neutrophils	0	0	$0–0.3 \times 10^3/\mu l$	$0–0.3 \times 10^9/L$
Lymphocytes	$0.8 \times 10^3/\mu l$ (8%)	$0.8 \times 10^9/L$ (8%)	$1.5–7.0 \times 10^3/\mu l$	$1.5–7.0 \times 10^9/L$
Monocytes	$0.6 \times 10^3/\mu l$ (7%)	$0.6 \times 10^9/L$ (7%)	$0–0.85 \times 10^3/\mu l$	$0–0.85 \times 10^9/L$
Eosinophils	$0 \times 10^3/\mu l$ (4%)	$0 \times 10^9/L$ (4%)	$0–0.75 \times 10^3/\mu l$	$0–0.75 \times 10^9/L$
Basophils	0	0	$0–0.2 \times 10^3/\mu l$	$0–0.2 \times 10^9/L$

MCH = mean corpuscular hemoglobin; MCHC = mean corpuscular hemoglobin concentration; MCV = mean corpuscular volume.

38. Serum Biochemical Profile

Analyte	Traditional Units	SI Units	Normal Values Traditional Units	Normal Values SI Units
Sodium	151 mEq/L	151 mmol/L	145–158 mEq/L	145–158 mmol/L
Potassium	4.6 mEq/L	4.6 mmol/L	3.6–5.8 mEq/L	3.6–5.8 mmol/L
Chloride	116 mEq/L	116 mmol/L	105–122 mEq/L	105–122 mmol/L
Calcium	10.8 mEq/L	2.69 mmol/L	9.0–11.8 mEq/L	2.24–2.95 mmol/L
Phosphorus	3.87 mEq/L	1.25 mmol/L	1.55–8.05 mEq/L	0.5–2.6 mmol/L
Urea	13.2 mg/dl	4.7 mmol/L	5.9–27.2 mg/dl	2.1–9.7 mmol/L
Creatinine	1.3 mg/dl	115 µmol/L	0.62–1.64 mg/dl	55–145 µmol/L
Glucose	93 mg/dl	5.2 mmol/L	60–158 mg/dl	3.3–8.7 mmol/L
Cholesterol	224 mg/dl	5.79 mmol/L	106–367 mg/dl	2.74–9.5 mmol/L
Total bilirubin	0.12 mg/dl	2 µmol/L	0–0.41 mg/dl	0–7 mmol/L
Amylase	851 IU/L	851 U/L	400–1800 IU/L	400–1800 U/L
ALP	66 IU/L	66 U/L	0–200 IU/L	0–200 U/L
AST	26 IU/L	26 U/L	10–50 IU/L	10–50 U/L
ALT	40 IU/L	40 U/L	0–130 IU/L	0–130 U/L
GGT	3 IU/L	3 U/L	0–6 IU/L	0–6 U/L
Creatine kinase	134 IU/L	134 U/L	0–460 IU/L	0–460 U/L
Total protein	6.4 g/dl	64 g/L	5.0–7.5 g/dl	50–75 g/L
Albumin	3.5 g/dl	35 g/L	2.2–3.5 g/dl	22–35 g/L
Globulins	2.9 g/dl	29 g/L	2.2–4.5 g/dl	22–45 g/L

ALT = alanine aminotransferase; ALP = alkaline phosphatase; AST = aspartate aminotransferase; GGT = γ-glutamyl transpeptidase.

39. Tensilon (edrophonium) response test: No response to edrophonium administration.

40. Ultrasound—cardiac: mild decrease in myocardial contractility (fractional shortening 22% [normal > 30%]; mild left atrial enlargement; mild left ventricular enlargement [increased end-diastolic and end-systolic dimensions]).

41. Ultrasound—abdominal: no abnormal findings

42. Urinalysis

Parameter	Result	Normal Values
Collection method	free flow	
Color/turbidity	yellow/clear	yellow/clear
Specific gravity	1.041	1.001–1.065
pH	6.0	4.5–8.5
Glucose	negative	negative
Ketones	negative	negative
Bilirubin	trace	trace to 1+
Occult blood	negative	negative
Protein	negative	negative to trace
RBC/high-power field	0–2	0–5
WBC/high-power field	0–3	0–5
Casts/low-power field	none	occasional hyaline
Epithelial cells/high-power field	none	occasional
Bacteria/high-power field	none	none
Crystals/high-power field	few phosphates	variable

pH = –log hydrogen ion concentration; RBC = red blood cell; WBC = white blood cell.

43. Urine culture: negative

44. Abdominocentesis: no fluid is obtained

45. Exploratory laparotomy: Cardiac arrest occurs during induction of general anesthesia. Cardiopulmonary resuscitation is unsuccessful.

46. Prothrombin time: 7.0 seconds (normal = 6.0–7.8 seconds)

47. Partial thromboplastin time: 18 seconds (normal = 11–21 seconds)

48. Mucosal bleeding time: 1.9 minutes (normal [dogs] = 1.7–4.2 minutes)

49. Fibrin degradation products: 5 μg/dl (normal = ≤ 20 μg/dl)

50. von Willebrand factor antigen: 95% (normal = 60%–152%)

51. Fecal flotation—routine: negative

52. Baermann fecal flotation: negative

53. Transtracheal wash: No abnormal findings. Aerobic bacterial culture is negative. Although this is a relatively noninvasive test, there are no clinical signs or test results warranting this procedure in this patient.

54. Gastroduodenoscopy—examination and biopsy: Cardiac arrest occurs during induction of general anesthesia. Cardiopulmonary resuscitation is unsuccessful.

55. Proctoscopy and colonoscopy—examination and biopsy: Cardiac arrest occurs during induction of general anesthesia. Cardiopulmonary resuscitation is unsuccessful.

56. Intestinal biopsy via laparotomy: Cardiac arrest occurs during induction of general anesthesia. Cardiopulmonary resuscitation is unsuccessful.

57. Bone marrow aspiration: normal

58. Lymph node needle aspirate: normal

59. Serum trypsin-like immunoreactivity: 8 μg/L (normal = 5–35 μg/L)

60. Splenoportogram: Cardiac arrest occurs during induction of general anesthesia. Cardiopulmonary resuscitation is unsuccessful.

61. Hepatic biopsy: Normal. There are no clinical signs or test results warranting this procedure in this patient.

62. Rhinotomy: Cardiac arrest occurs during induction of general anesthesia. Cardiopulmonary resuscitation is unsuccessful.

63. Fundoscopic examination: no abnormal findings

64. Feline leukemia virus (serum enzyme-linked immunosorbent assay [ELISA]): Negative. The laboratory technician asks why you are performing this test on a dog.

65. Feline immunodeficiency virus (serum enzyme-linked immunosorbent assay [ELISA]): Negative. The laboratory technician asks why you are performing this test on a dog.

66. Feline infectious peritonitis virus titer: No measurable titer. The laboratory technician asks why you are performing this test on a dog.

67. Ehrlichia canis titer: negative

68. Rocky Mountain spotted fever titer: < 1:64 (active infection is unlikely with titers ≤ 1:64)

69. Cryptococcal capsular antigen (serum): negative

70. Aspergillus titer: negative

71. Toxoplasma titer:
    IgG = no measurable titer
    IgM = no measurable titer

72. Survey radiographs—nasal series: No abnormal findings. Cardiac arrest occurs while the animal is under general anesthesia. Cardiopulmonary resuscitation is unsuccessful.

73. Rhinoscopy—examination and biopsy: No abnormal findings. Cardiac arrest occurs while the animal is under general anesthesia. Cardiopulmonary resuscitation is unsuccessful.

74. Traumatic nasal flush: No abnormal findings. Cardiac arrest occurs while the animal is under general anesthesia. Cardiopulmonary resuscitation is unsuccessful.

75. Thoracocentesis: No fluid is obtained.

76. Fine-needle aspirate of mass: No masses are identified in this patient.

77. Fundoscopic examination: no abnormal findings

78. Serum cobalamin: 530 ng/L (normal = 200–1680 ng/L)

79. Serum folate: 16.2 μg/L (normal = 13.4–38 ug/L)

80. Fat absorption test: normal

81. N-benzoyl-L-tyrosyl-para-aminobenzoic Acid (BT PABA) Digestion Test

Interval	Serum PABA (μg/dl) *	
	Patient	Normal Values
0	0	39 ± 15
30 minutes	489	500 ± 152
60 minutes	571	670 ± 140
90 minutes	654	637 ± 124
120 minutes	555	560 ± 116

* Peak < 100 μg/dl = exocrine pancreatic insufficiency; peak > 300 μg/dl = normal exocrine pancreatic function.
PABA = para-aminobenzoic acid.

82. 6 hour urine para-aminobenzoic acid (PABA) excretion: 61% of administered dose (normal = 63±4% of administered dose)

83. Xylose Absorption Test

Interval	Plasma Xylose (mg/dl)
0	2
1 hour	61
2 hours	42
3 hours	21
4 hours	15

> 45 mg/dl at 1 hour is normal.

84. Fecal culture: No pathogens grown.

85. Duodenal aspirate culture: 6×10^4 microorganisms/ml (normal < 10^5 microorganisms/ml)

86. Blood ammonia: 22 μmol/L (normal = 10–82 μmol/L)

87. Ammonia Tolerance Test

Parameter	Result	Normal Values
Fasting ammonia	22 μmol/L	10–82 μmol/L
Post-challenge ammonia	51 μmol/L	10–82 μmol/L

88. Serum osmolality: 310 mOsm/kg (normal = 295–315 mOsm/kg)

89. Serum protein electrophoresis: normal

90. Coomb's test: negative

91. Basal endogenous adrenocorticotropic hormone (ACTH) concentration: 20.2 pmol/L [92 pg/ml] (< 4.4 pmol/L [20 pg/ml]—consistent with an adrenal tumor in a dog with known hyperadrenocorticism; >9.9 pmol/L [45 pg/ml]—consistent with pituitary dependent hyperadrenocorticism in a dog with known hyperadrenocorticism)

92. Endogenous parathyroid hormone concentration: 3.5 pmol/L (normal = 2–13 pmol/L [dogs]; 0–4 pmol/L [cats])

93. Endogenous thyroid stimulating hormone (TSH) concentration: 0.21 ng/ml (normal = 0.06–0.32 ng/ml)

94. Urine cortisol:creatinine ratio: 6.5 × 10^{-6} (normal < 10 × 10^{-6})

95. Bronchoscopy—examination and sampling: The dog goes into cardiac arrest during anesthetic induction and cannot be resuscitated.

96. Rectal scraping cytology: no abnormalities

97. Fluoroscopy—thorax: normal

98. Fluoroscopy—gastric (in conjunction with upper gastrointestinal [GI] contrast study): normal

99. Thoracotomy: Cardiac arrest occurs during induction of general anesthesia. Cardiopulmonary resuscitation is unsuccessful.

100. Urine protein:creatinine ratio: 0.2 (normal < 1.0)

101. Distemper virus—cytology of conjunctival scraping: negative

102. Coronavirus—Electron microscopy (EM) on feces: negative

103. Parvovirus—Electron microscopy (EM) on feces: negative

104. Parvovirus—enzyme-linked immunosorbent assay (ELISA) on feces: negative

105. Pericardiocentesis: Fresh blood is obtained and ventricular tachycardia is induced because there is no pericardial effusion and the heart has been punctured.

106. Adrenocorticotropic Hormone (ACTH) Stimulation Test

Parameter	Result	Normal Values
Baseline cortisol	140 nmol/L (5.2 μg/dl)	25–125 nmol/L (0.91–4.5 μg/dl)
Post-ACTH cortisol	860 nmol/L (31.9 μg/dl)	200–550 nmol/L (7.2–20 μg/dl)

ACTH = adrenocorticotropic hormone.

107. Arterial Blood Gas Analysis

Parameter	Result	Normal Values
pH	7.29	7.351–7.463
PCO_2	36 mmHg	30.8–42.8 mmHg
PO_2	94 mmHg	80.9–103.3 mmHg
HCO_3^-	16.9 mEq/L (mmol/L)	18.8–25.6 mEq/L

HCO_3^- = bicarbonate; PCO_2 = partial pressure of carbon dioxide; pH = −log hydrogen ion concentration; PO_2 = partial pressure of oxygen.

108. Bile Acid Concentrations

Parameter	Result	Normal Values
Fasting	35.2 mg/L (88 μmol/L)	< 4 mg/L (< 10 μmol/L)
2-hour postprandial	49.6 mg/L (124 μmol/L)	< 8 mg/L (< 20 μmol/L)

109. Endogenous creatinine clearance: 2.4 ml/min/kg (normal = 2.3 ± 0.5 ml/min/kg)

110. Cardiac catheterization: Mild to moderate regurgitation noted across the mitral valve. No other abnormalities are noted. There are no indications warranting this invasive procedure in this patient.

111. Cerebrospinal fluid collection and analysis: The animal goes into cardiac arrest during induction of anesthesia. Cardiopulmonary resuscitation is unsuccessful.

112. Complete Blood Count

Parameter	Traditional Units	SI Units	Normal Values Traditional Units	Normal Values SI Units
Hemoglobin	13.6 g/dl	136 g/L	13.2–19.2 g/dl	132–193 g/L
Hematocrit	30%	0.30 L/L	38–57%	0.38–0.57 L/L
Erythrocytes	$4.62 \times 10^6/\mu l$	$4.62 \times 10^{12}/L$	$5.6–8.5 \times 10^6/\mu l$	$5.6–8.5 \times 10^{12}/L$
MCV	64.9 mm^3	64.9 fl	62–71 mm^3	62–71 fl
MCH	24 pg	24 pg	22–25 pg	22–25 pg
MCHC	37.0%	370 g/L	33.7–36.5%	337–365 g/L
Reticulocytes	0.3%	0.3%	0–1.5%	0–1.5%
Platelets	$110 \times 10^3/\mu l$	$110 \times 10^9/L$	$145–440 \times 10^3/\mu l$	$145–440 \times 10^9/L$
Total nucleated cell count	$15.3 \times 10^3/\mu l$	$15.3 \times 10^9/L$	$6.1–17.4 \times 10^3/\mu l$	$6.1–17.4 \times 10^9/L$
Neutrophils	$13.5 \times 10^3/\mu l$ (89%)	$13.5 \times 10^9/L$ (89%)	$3.9–12 \times 10^3/\mu l$	$3.9–12 \times 10^9/L$
Band neutrophils	0.3 (2%)	0.3 (2%)	$0–1.0 \times 10^3/\mu l$	$0–1.0 \times 10^9/L$
Lymphocytes	$0.5 \times 10^3/\mu l$ (3%)	$0.5 \times 10^9/L$ (3%)	$0.8–3.6 \times 10^3/\mu l$	$0.8–3.6 \times 10^9/L$
Monocytes	$0.8 \times 10^3/\mu l$ (5%)	$0.8 \times 10^9/L$ (5%)	$0–1.8 \times 10^3/\mu l$	$0–1.8 \times 10^9/L$
Eosinophils	$0.2 \times 10^3/\mu l$ (1%)	$0.2 \times 10^9/L$ (1%)	$0–1.9 \times 10^3/\mu l$	$0–1.9 \times 10^9/L$
Basophils	0	0	$0–0.2 \times 10^3/\mu l$	$0–0.2 \times 10^9/L$

MCH = mean corpuscular hemoglobin; MCHC = mean corpuscular hemoglobin concentration; MCV = mean corpuscular volume.

113. Computerized tomography—skull: The animal goes into cardiac arrest during induction of anesthesia. Cardiopulmonary resuscitation is unsuccessful.

114. Computerized tomography—abdomen: complex mass (approximately 5 cm × 8 cm [2″ × 3″]) on the spleen

115. Contrast radiographs—myelogram: The animal goes into cardiac arrest during induction of anesthesia. Cardiopulmonary resuscitation is unsuccessful.

116. Contrast radiographs—diskogram (lumbosacral): The animal goes into cardiac arrest during induction of anesthesia. Cardiopulmonary resuscitation is unsuccessful.

117. Contrast radiographs—epidurogram: The animal goes into cardiac arrest during induction of anesthesia. Cardiopulmonary resuscitation is unsuccessful.

118. Contrast radiographs—cystogram: A mass lesion/irregular bladder wall is seen in the trigone area.

119. Contrast radiographs—upper gastrointestinal study: thickened small intestinal walls

120. Contrast radiographs—intravenous pyelogram: Following the procedure the dog goes into acute renal failure because of the pre-existing hypovolemia and reduced renal perfusion.

121. Electrocardiogram: normal

122. Electromyography: The animal goes into cardiac arrest during induction of anesthesia. Cardiopulmonary resuscitation is unsuccessful.

123. Fasting serum insulin concentration: 185 pmol/L [25.7 μU/ml] (normal = 35–200 pmol/L [4.9—27.9 μU/ml])

124. Low-Dose Dexamethasone Response Test

Parameter	Result	Normal Values
Baseline cortisol	100 nmol/L (3.7 μg/dl)	25–125 nmol/L (0.91–4.5 μg/dl)
4–hour cortisol	14 nmol/L (0.5 μg/dl)	
8–hour cortisol	54 nmol/L (2.0 μg/dl)	< 40 nmol/L (< 1.4 μg/dl)

125. High-Dose Dexamethasone Response Test

Parameter	Result	Normal Values
Baseline cortisol	115 nmol/L (4.2 μg/dl)	25–125 nmol/L (0.91–4.5 μg/dl)
4–hour cortisol	11 nmol/L (0.42 μg/dl)	
8–hour cortisol	35 nmol/L (1.3 μg/dl)	< 50% of baseline = pituitary dependent hyperadrenocorticism in a dog with known hyperadrenocorticism

126. Glucose tolerance test: Normal. Although this is a non-invasive test, it would add to the patient's diagnostic costs and is not needed in a dog with an insignificant increase in serum glucose. A serum glucose at the level seen in this dog will not cause or contribute to the polyuria.

127. Water deprivation/vasopressin response test: The signs of shock worsen in this dog.

128. Muscle biopsy—left cranial tibialis muscle: No abnormal findings. Excessive hemorrhage occurs during and after the biopsy procedure.

129. Nerve conduction studies: The animal goes into cardiac arrest during induction of anesthesia. Cardiopulmonary resuscitation is unsuccessful.

130. Neurologic examination:
Cranial nerves: normal
Spinal reflexes (patellar, withdrawal, perineal): normal
Conscious proprioception: difficult to determine because of the dog's weakness and inability to stand
No areas of hyperpathia, pain, or muscle atrophy

131. Peripheral nerve biopsy—right distal peroneal nerve: No abnormal findings. There is excessive hemorrhage during and after the procedure.

132. Survey radiographs—thoracic: no abnormal findings

133. Survey radiographs—abdominal: Abdominal detail is somewhat obscured by fluid in the abdomen. The spleen is enlarged and irregular in shape.

134. Survey radiographs—cervical spine: no abnormal findings

135. Survey radiographs—thoracolumbar spine: no abnormal findings

136. Survey radiographs—lumbosacral spine: no abnormal findings

137. Baseline serum T_4 (thyroxine) concentration: 8 nmol/L (0.6 μg/dl) Normal values = 12–50 nmol/L (0.9–3.9 μg/dl)

138. Serum Biochemical Profile

Analyte	Traditional Units	SI Units	Normal Values Traditional Units	Normal Values SI Units
Sodium	149 mEq/L	149 mmol/L	145–158 mEq/L	145–158 mmol/L
Potassium	3.7 mEq/L	3.7 mmol/L	3.6–5.8 mEq/L	3.6–5.8 mmol/L
Chloride	115 mEq/L	115 mmol/L	105–122 mEq/L	105–122 mmol/L
Calcium	9.6 mEq/L	2.4 mmol/L	9.0–11.8 mEq/L	2.24–2.95 mmol/L
Phosphorus	3.1 mEq/L	1.0 mmol/L	1.55–8.05 mEq/L	0.5–2.6 mmol/L
Urea	8.4 mg/dl	3.0 mmol/L	5.9–27.2 mg/dl	2.1–9.7 mmol/L
Creatinine	0.83 mg/dl	73 μmol/L	0.62–1.64 mg/dl	55–145 μmol/L
Glucose	119 mg/dl	6.6 mmol/L	60–158 mg/dl	3.3–8.7 mmol/L
Cholesterol	173 mg/dl	4.46 mmol/L	106–367 mg/dl	2.74–9.5 mmol/L
Total bilirubin	0 mg/dl	0 μmol/L	0–0.41 mg/dl	0–7 mmol/L
Amylase	858 IU/L	858 U/L	400–1800 IU/L	400–1800 U/L
ALP	85 IU/L	85 U/L	0–200 IU/L	0–200 U/L
AST	49 IU/L	49 U/L	10–50 IU/L	10–50 U/L
ALT	16 IU/L	16 U/L	0–130 IU/L	0–130 U/L
GGT	1 IU/L	1 U/L	0–6 IU/L	0–6 U/L
Creatine kinase	231 IU/L	231 U/L	0–460 IU/L	0–460 U/L
Total protein	5.3 g/dl	53 g/L	5.0–7.5 g/dl	50–75 g/L
Albumin	2.2 g/dl	22 g/L	2.2–3.5 g/dl	22–35 g/L
Globulins	3.1 g/dl	31 g/L	2.2–4.5 g/dl	22–45 g/L

ALT = alanine aminotransferase; ALP = alkaline phosphatase; AST = aspartate aminotransferase; GGT = γ-glutamyl transpeptidase.

139. Ultrasound—cardiac: regurgitation associated with mitral valve incompetence; mild increase in left atrial size

140. Ultrasound—abdominal: complex mass (approximately 5 cm × 8 cm [2″ × 3″]) of mixed echogenicity associated with the spleen; moderate amount of free fluid within the abdomen

141. Urinalysis

Parameter	Result	Normal Values
Collection method	free flow	
Color/turbidity	yellow/clear	yellow/clear
Specific gravity	1.041	1.001–1.065
pH	6.0	4.5–8.5
Glucose	negative	negative
Ketones	negative	negative
Bilirubin	trace	trace to 1+
Occult blood	positive	negative
Protein	1+	negative to trace
RBC/high-power field	40–50	0–5
WBC/high-power field	0–3	0–5
Casts/low-power field	none	occasional hyaline
Epithelial cells/high-power field	none	occasional
Bacteria/high-power field	occasional	none
Crystals/high-power field	none	variable

pH = –log hydrogen ion concentation; RBC = red blood cell; WBC = white blood cell.

142. Urine culture: low numbers (< 100 cfu/ml) of *Escherichia coli*

143. Abdominocentesis:
Appearance: grossly bloody
Nucleated cell count: $5.6 \times 10^3/\mu l$ ($5.6 \times 10^9/L$)
Red blood cell count: $3.8 \times 10^6/\mu l$ ($3.8 \times 10^{12}/L$)
Hematocrit: 25% (0.25L/L)
Protein: 4.5 g/dl (45 g/L)
Specific gravity: 1.027
Cytologic description: numerous erythrocytes and moderate numbers of mesothelial cells, macrophages, small lymphocytes, and nondegenerate neutrophils; moderate numbers of macrophages contain hemosiderin pigment or demonstrate erythrocytophagia.

144. Exploratory laparotomy: A large 5 cm × 8 cm (2″ × 3″) dark red friable mass is associated with the spleen. There is abundant free blood with blood clots in the abdominal cavity. There are no visible metastases to other intra-abdominal organs. Histopathologic examination of the splenic mass reveals hemangiosarcoma.

145. Prothrombin time: 8 seconds (normal = 7–11 seconds)

146. Partial thromboplastin time: 19 seconds (normal = 13–20 seconds)

147. Mucosal bleeding time: 9.0 minutes (normal = 1.7–4.2 minutes)

148. Baermann fecal flotation: positive. Numerous L1 larvae present and identified as *Crenosoma vulpis* (fox lungworm).

149. Transtracheal wash: No abnormal findings. Aerobic bacterial culture is negative. The puncture site over the trachea seems to bleed excessively.

150. Gastroduodenoscopy—examination and biopsy: No abnormal findings. There are no clinical signs or test results warranting this procedure in this patient.

151. Proctoscopy and colonoscopy—examination and biopsy: No abnormal findings. There are no clinical signs or test results warranting this procedure in this patient.

152. Intestinal biopsy via laparotomy: No abnormal findings

153. Bone marrow aspiration: megakaryocytic hyperplasia; erythroid and myeloid cell lines appear normal

154. Lymph node needle aspirate: Cytologic evaluation reveals reactive hyperplasia.

155. Serum trypsin-like immunoreactivity: normal

156. Splenoportogram: Normal. There are no clinical signs or test results warranting this procedure in this patient.

157. Hepatic biopsy: Normal. The dog seems to bleed excessively after the procedure.

158. Rhinotomy: No abnormal findings. There are no clinical signs or test results warranting this invasive procedure in this patient.

159. Fundoscopic examination: Several small pinpoint retinal hemorrhages are observed in both eyes.

160. Feline leukemia virus (serum enzyme-linked immunosorbent assay [ELISA]): positive

161. Feline immunodeficiency virus (serum enzyme-linked immunosorbent assay [ELISA]): negative.

162. Feline infectious peritonitis virus titer: negative

163. *Ehrlichia canis* titer: Negative. The laboratory technician asks why you are performing this test on a cat.

164. Rocky Mountain spotted fever titer: <1:16 (active infection is unlikely with titers ≤ 1:64)

165. Cryptococcal capsular antigen (serum): positive

166. Toxoplasma titer:
IgG = 1:32
IgM = no measurable titer

167. Survey radiographs—nasal series: There is a moderate increased opacity in the right nasal cavity. Significant turbinate destruction is not visible.

168. Rhinoscopy—examination and biopsy: The right nasal cavity is blood-filled, with no obvious masses, foreign bodies, or mucosal inflammation. The left nasal cavity appears normal. The dog bleeds excessively following biopsy and requires a blood transfusion. Biopsy results are normal.

169. Traumatic nasal flush: No abnormal findings. The dog bleeds excessively following biopsy and requires a blood transfusion.

170. Thoracocentesis:
Appearance: pale yellow, cloudy
Nucleated cell count: $14.2 \times 10^3/\mu l$ ($14.2 \times 10^9/L$)
Protein: 3.6 g/dl (36 g/L)
Specific gravity: 1.022
Cytologic description: nucleated cells are comprised primarily (91%) of large lymphoblasts with the remaining nucleated cells composed of approximately equal numbers of macrophages, neutrophils, and small lymphocytes; consistent with lymphosarcoma.

171. Fine-needle aspirate of mass— aspirate of cranial mediastinal mass: Majority of cells are large lymphoblasts; consistent with lymphosarcoma.

172. Serum cobalamin: 184 ng/L (normal = 225–660 ng/L)

173. Serum folate: 5.5 μg/L (normal = 6.7–17.4 μg/L)

174. Fat absorption test: Minimal lipemia after a meal of food and vegetable oil; minimal lipemia after a meal of food, vegetable oil, and pancreatic enzymes.

175. N-benzoyl-L-tyrosol-para-aminobenzoic Acid (BT PABA) Digestion Test

	Serum PABA (μg/dl) *	
Interval	Patient	Normal Values
0	0	39 ± 15
30 minutes	284	500 ± 152
60 minutes	361	670 ± 140
90 minutes	524	637 ± 124
120 minutes	403	560 ± 116

* Peak < 100 μg/dl = exocrine pancreatic insufficiency; peak > 300 μg/dl = normal exocrine pancreatic function.
PABA = para-aminobenzoic acid.

176. 6-hour urine para-aminobenzoic acid (PABA) excretion: 59% of administered dose (normal = 63±4% of administered dose)

177. Xylose Absorption Test

Interval	Plasma Xylose (mg/dl)
0	3
1 hour	35
2 hours	32
3 hours	21
4 hours	15

> 45 mg/dl at 1 hour is normal.

178. Duodenal aspirate culture: The animal goes into cardiac arrest during induction of general anesthesia. Cardiopulmonary resuscitation is unsuccessful.

179. Blood ammonia: 140 μmol/L (normal = 10–82 μmol/L)

180. Ammonia Tolerance Test

Parameter	Result	Normal Values
Fasting ammonia	140 μmol/L	10–82 μmol/L
Post-challenge ammonia	200 μmol/L	10–82 μmol/L

The dog becomes very depressed and has three seizures.

181. Serum Biochemical Profile

Analyte	Traditional Units	SI Units	Normal Values Traditional Units	Normal Values SI Units
Sodium	140 mEq/L	140 mmol/L	145–158 mEq/L	145–158 mmol/L
Potassium	11.0 mEq/L	11.0 mmol/L	3.6–5.8 mEq/L	3.6–5.8 mmol/L
Chloride	101 mEq/L	101 mmol/L	105–122 mEq/L	105–122 mmol/L
Calcium	9.3 mEq/L	2.32 mmol/L	9.0–11.8 mEq/L	2.24–2.95 mmol/L
Phosphorus	11.7 mEq/L	3.78 mmol/L	1.55–8.05 mEq/L	0.5–2.6 mmol/L
Urea	121 mg/dl	43.2 mmol/L	5.9–27.2 mg/dl	2.1–9.7 mmol/L
Creatinine	5.8 mg/dl	513 μmol/L	0.62–1.64 mg/dl	55–145 μmol/L
Glucose	69 mg/dl	3.8 mmol/L	60–158 mg/dl	3.3–8.7 mmol/L
Cholesterol	132 mg/dl	3.4 mmol/L	106–367 mg/dl	2.74–9.5 mmol/L
Total bilirubin	0.18 mg/dl	3 μmol/L	0–0.41 mg/dl	0–7 mmol/L
Amylase	922 IU/L	922 U/L	400–1800 IU/L	400–1800 U/L
ALP	78 IU/L	78 U/L	0–200 IU/L	0–200 U/L
AST	15 IU/L	15 U/L	10–50 IU/L	10–50 U/L
ALT	22 IU/L	22 U/L	0–130 IU/L	0–130 U/L
GGT	4 IU/L	4 U/L	0–6 IU/L	0–6 U/L
Creatine kinase	237 IU/L	237 U/L	0–460 IU/L	0–460 U/L
Total protein	8.2 g/dl	82 g/L	5.0–7.5 g/dl	50–75 g/L
Albumin	4.1 g/dl	41 g/L	2.2–3.5 g/dl	22–35 g/L
Globulins	4.1 g/dl	41 g/L	2.2–4.5 g/dl	22–45 g/L

ALT = alanine aminotransferase; ALP = alkaline phosphatase; AST = aspartate aminotransferase; GGT = γ-glutamyl transpeptidase.

182. Urinalysis

Parameter	Result	Normal Values
Collection method	cystocentesis	
Color/turbidity	pale yellow/clear	yellow/clear
Specific gravity	1.015	1.001–1.065
pH	6.0	4.5–8.5
Glucose	negative	negative
Ketones	negative	negative
Bilirubin	trace	trace to 1+
Occult blood	negative	negative
Protein	negative	negative to trace
RBC/high-power field	0–1	0–5
WBC/high-power field	0–1	0–5
Casts/low-power field	none	occasional hyaline
Epithelial cells/high-power field	none	occasional
Bacteria/high-power field	none	none
Crystals/high-power field	none	variable

pH = −log hydrogen ion concentration; RBC = red blood cell; WBC = white blood cell.

183. Exploratory laparotomy: The uterus is markedly enlarged, hyperemic, and fluid-filled.

184. Complete Blood Count

Parameter	Traditional Units	SI Units	Normal Values Traditional Units	Normal Values SI Units
Hemoglobin	15 g/dl	150 g/L	13.2–19.2 g/dl	132–193 g/L
Hematocrit	40.8%	0.408 L/L	38–57%	0.38–0.57 L/L
Erythrocytes	$6.01 \times 10^6/\mu l$	$6.01 \times 10^{12}/L$	$5.6–8.5 \times 10^6/\mu l$	$5.6–8.5 \times 10^{12}/L$
MCV	67.9 mm³	67.9 fl	62–71 mm³	62–71 fl
MCH	25 pg	25 pg	22–25 pg	22–25 pg
MCHC	365%	365 g/L	33.7–36.5%	337–365 g/L
Reticulocytes	0%	0%	0–1.5%	0–1.5%
Platelets	$200 \times 10^3/\mu l$	$200 \times 10^9/L$	$145–440 \times 10^3/\mu l$	$145–440 \times 10^9/L$
Total nucleated cell count	$44.5 \times 10^3/\mu l$	$44.5 \times 10^9/L$	$6.1–17.4 \times 10^3/\mu l$	$6.1–17.4 \times 10^9/L$
Neutrophils	$36.0 \times 10^3/\mu l$ (81%) 1^+ toxicity	$36.0 \times 10^9/L$ (81%)	$3.9–12 \times 10^3/\mu l$	$3.9–12 \times 10^9/L$
Band neutrophils	$4.4 \times 10^3/\mu l$ (10%)	$4.5 \times 10^3/L$ (10%)	$0–1.0 \times 10^3/\mu l$	$0–1.0 \times 10^9/L$
Lymphocytes	$0.9 \times 10^3/\mu l$ (2%)	$0.9 \times 10^9/L$ (2%)	$0.8–3.6 \times 10^3/\mu l$	$0.8–3.6 \times 10^9/L$
Monocytes	$3.1 \times 10^3/\mu l$ (7%)	$3.1 \times 10^9/L$ (7%)	$0–1.8 \times 10^3/\mu l$	$0–1.8 \times 10^9/L$
Eosinophils	0	0	$0–1.9 \times 10^3/\mu l$	$0–1.9 \times 10^9/L$
Basophils	0	0	$0–0.2 \times 10^3/\mu l$	$0–0.2 \times 10^9/L$

MCH = mean corpuscular hemoglobin; MCHC = mean corpuscular hemoglobin concentration; MCV = mean corpuscular volume.

185. Urinalysis

Parameter	Result	Normal Values
Collection method	cystocentesis	
Color/turbidity	yellow/clear	yellow/clear
Specific gravity	1.022	1.001–1.065
pH	6.0	4.5–8.5
Glucose	negative	negative
Ketones	negative	negative
Bilirubin	trace	trace to 1+
Occult blood	negative	negative
Protein	negative	negative to trace
RBC/high-power field	0–5	0–5
WBC/high-power field	0–3	0–5
Casts/low-power field	none	occasional hyaline
Epithelial cells/high-power field	none	occasional
Bacteria/high-power field	none	none
Crystals/high-power field	none	variable

pH = −log hydrogen ion concentration; RBC = red blood cell; WBC = white blood cell.

186. Serum Biochemical Profile

Analyte	Traditional Units	SI Units	Normal Values Traditional Units	Normal Values SI Units
Sodium	155 mEq/L	155 mmol/L	145–158 mEq/L	145–158 mmol/L
Potassium	3.6 mEq/L	3.6 mmol/L	3.6–5.8 mEq/L	3.6–5.8 mmol/L
Chloride	118 mEq/L	118 mmol/L	105–122 mEq/L	105–122 mmol/L
Calcium	9.3 mEq/L	2.32 mmol/L	9.0–11.8 mEq/L	2.24–2.95 mmol/L
Phosphorus	8.0 mEq/L	2.6 mmol/L	1.55–8.05 mEq/L	0.5–2.6 mmol/L
Urea	26 mg/dl	9.3 mmol/L	5.9–27.2 mg/dl	2.1–9.7 mmol/L
Creatinine	1.55 mg/dl	137 µmol/L	0.62–1.64 mg/dl	55–145 µmol/L
Glucose	106 mg/dl	5.9 mmol/L	60–158 mg/dl	3.3–8.7 mmol/L
Cholesterol	132 mg/dl	3.4 mmol/L	106–367 mg/dl	2.74–9.5 mmol/L
Total bilirubin	0.18 mg/dl	3 µmol/L	0–0.41 mg/dl	0–7 mmol/L
Amylase	922 IU/L	922 U/L	400–1800 IU/L	400–1800 U/L
ALP	75 IU/L	75 U/L	0–200 IU/L	0–200 U/L
AST	42 IU/L	42 U/L	10–50 IU/L	10–50 U/L
ALT	63 IU/L	63 U/L	0–130 IU/L	0–130 U/L
GGT	4 IU/L	4 U/L	0–6 IU/L	0–6 U/L
Creatine kinase	237 IU/L	237 U/L	0–460 IU/L	0–460 U/L
Total protein	7.1 g/dl	71 g/L	5.0–7.5 g/dl	50–75 g/L
Albumin	2.8 g/dl	28 g/L	2.2–3.5 g/dl	22–35 g/L
Globulins	4.3 g/dl	43 g/L	2.2–4.5 g/dl	22–45 g/L

ALT = alanine aminotransferase; ALP = alkaline phosphatase; AST = aspartate aminotransferase; GGT = γ-glutamyl transpeptidase.

187. Urinalysis

Parameter	Result	Normal Values
Collection method	cystocentesis	
Color/turbidity	yellow/clear	yellow/clear
Specific gravity	1.015	1.001–1.065
pH	6.0	4.5–8.5
Glucose	negative	negative
Ketones	negative	negative
Bilirubin	trace	trace to 1+
Occult blood	negative	negative
Protein	negative	negative to trace
RBC/high-power field	0–2	0–5
WBC/high-power field	0–3	0–5
Casts/low-power field	none	occasional hyaline
Epithelial cells/high-power field	none	occasional
Bacteria/high-power field	none	none
Crystals/high-power field	none	variable

pH = –log hydrogen ion concentration; RBC = red blood cell; WBC = white blood cell.

188. Survey radiographs—thoracic: microcardia and a narrowed vena cava cranial to the diaphragm

189. Distemper virus—cytology of conjunctival scraping: Negative. The laboratory technician asks why you are performing this test on a cat.

190. Serum osmolality : 349 mOsm/kg (normal = 295–315 mOsm/kg)

191. Basal endogenous adrenocorticotropic hormone (ACTH) concentration: 22.7 pmol/L [103 pg/ml] (< 4.4 pmol/L [20 pg/ml]—consistent with an adrenal tumor in a dog with known hyperadrenocorticism; > 9.9 pmol/L [45 pg/ml]—consistent with pituitary-dependent hyperadrenocorticism in a dog with known hyperadrenocorticism)

192. Urine cortisol:creatinine ratio: 12.1 × 10^{-6} (normal < 10 × 10^{-6})

193. Bronchoscopy—examination and sampling: normal

194. Fluoroscopy—thorax: A cranial mediastinal mass is visualized.

195. Fluoroscopy—gastric (in conjunction with upper gastrointestinal [GI] contrast study): The upper GI contrast study has to be discontinued because of increased weakness and bradycardia.

196. Thoracotomy: The dog develops severe hemorrhage during surgery and dies despite fluid therapy and a blood transfusion.

197. Pericardiocentesis: You obtain fresh blood and induce a paroxysm of ventricular tachycardia because there is no pericardial effusion and you have punctured the heart. Hemorrhage continues into the pericardial sac and the dog develops acute cardiac tamponade and dies.

198. Adrenocorticotropic Hormone (ACTH) Stimulation Test

Parameter	Result	Normal Values
Baseline cortisol	5 nmol/L (0.18 μg/dl)	25–125 nmol/L (0.91–4.5 μg/dl)
Post-ACTH cortisol	7 nmol/L (0.26 μg/dl)	200–550 nmol/L (7.2–20 μg/dl)

199. Arterial Blood Gas Analysis

Parameter	Result	Normal Values
pH	7.32	7.310–7.462
PCO_2	36 mmHg	25.2–36.8 mmHg
PO_2	94 mmHg	95.4–118.2 mmHg
HCO_3^-	18 mEq/L (mmol/L)	14.4–21.6 mEq/L

HCO_3^- = bicarbonate; PCO_2 = partial pressure of carbon dioxide; pH = –log hydrogen ion concentration; PO_2 = partial pressure of oxygen.

200. Cardiac catheterization: Normal. In this case there are no clinical signs or other test results warranting this invasive procedure.

201. Cerebrospinal Fluid Collection and Analysis

Parameter	Result	Normal Values
Protein	0.32 g/L (32 mg/dl)	0.10–0.30 g/L (10–30 mg/dl)
Nucleated cells	0.043×10^9/L (43/mm³)	$0.0–0.002 \times 10^9$/L (0–2/mm³)

Cellularity is high and consists primarily of mononuclear cells with increased numbers of neutrophils and occasional eosinophils. Several yeast organisms consistent with *Cryptococcus* species are observed.

202. Complete Blood Count

Parameter	Traditional Units	SI Units	Normal Values Traditional Units	Normal Values SI Units
Hemoglobin	14.2 g/dl	142 g/L	13.2–19.2 g/dl	132–193 g/L
Hematocrit	40%	0.40 L/L	38–57%	0.38–0.57 L/L
Erythrocytes	5.67×10^6/µl	5.67×10^{12}/L	$5.6–8.5 \times 10^6$/µl	$5.6–8.5 \times 10^{12}$/L
MCV	70.2 mm³	70.2 fl	62–71 mm³	62–71 fl
MCH	25 pg	25 pg	22–25 pg	22–25 pg
MCHC	35.7%	357 g/L	33.7–36.5%	337–365 g/L
Reticulocytes	0.1%	0.1%	0–1.5%	0–1.5%
Platelets	6×10^3/µl	6×10^9/L	$145–440 \times 10^3$/µl	$145–440 \times 10^9$/L
Total nucleated cell count	8.9×10^3/µl	8.9×10^9/L	$6.1–17.4 \times 10^3$/µl	$6.1–17.4 \times 10^9$/L
Neutrophils	6.3×10^3/µl (71%)	6.3×10^9/L (71%)	$3.9–12 \times 10^3$/µl	$3.9–12 \times 10^9$/L
Band neutrophils	0	0	$0–1.0 \times 10^3$/µl	$0–1.0 \times 10^9$/L
Lymphocytes	1.7×10^3/µl (19%)	1.7×10^9/L (19%)	$0.8–3.6 \times 10^3$/µl	$0.8–3.6 \times 10^9$/L
Monocytes	0.5×10^3/µl (6%)	0.5×10^9/L (6%)	$0–1.8 \times 10^3$/µl	$0–1.8 \times 10^9$/L
Eosinophils	0.4×10^3/µl (4%)	0.4×10^9/L (4%)	$0–1.9 \times 10^3$/µl	$0–1.9 \times 10^9$/L
Basophils	0	0	$0–0.2 \times 10^3$/µl	$0–0.2 \times 10^9$/L

MCH = mean corpuscular hemoglobin; MCHC = mean corpuscular hemoglobin concentration; MCV = mean corpuscular volume.

203. Computerized tomography—skull: Normal. The dog has a prolonged recovery from anesthesia.

204. Computerized tomography of the abdomen shows bilateral adrenomegaly and mild hepatomegaly.

205. Contrast radiographs—myelogram: Normal. The dog has an adverse reaction to the contrast material (i.e., severe seizure activity following the procedure) caused by inflammation in the CNS.

206. Contrast radiographs—diskogram (lumbosacral): Normal. There are no clinical indications warranting such an invasive diagnostic procedure in this animal. The dog has a prolonged recovery from anesthesia.

207. Contrast radiographs—epidurogram: Normal. There are no clinical indications warranting such an invasive diagnostic procedure in this animal. The dog has a prolonged recovery from anesthesia.

208. Contrast radiographs—cystogram: The dog goes into cardiac arrest during induction of anesthesia. Cardiopulmonary resuscitation is unsuccesful.

209. Contrast radiographs—upper gastrointestinal (GI) study: Procedure discontinued because of worsening shock and bradycardia.

210. Electrocardiogram: T waves are tall and peaked; P waves are absent

211. Low-Dose Dexamethasone Response Test

Parameter	Result	Normal Values
Baseline cortisol	3 nmol/L (0 μg/dl)	25–125 nmol/L (0.91–4.5 μg/dl)
4–hour cortisol	0 nmol/L (0 μg/dl)	
8–hour cortisol	0 nmol/L (0 μg/dl)	< 40 nmol/L (< 1.4 μg/dl)

212. High-Dose Dexamethasone Response Test

Parameter	Result	Normal Values
Baseline cortisol	3 nmol/L (0 μg/dl)	25–125 nmol/L (0.91–4.5 μg/dl)
4–hour cortisol	0 nmol/L (0 μg/dl)	
8–hour cortisol	0 nmol/L (0 μg/dl)	< 50% of baseline = pituitary dependent hyperadrenocorticism in a dog with known hyperadrenocorticism

213. Water deprivation/vasopressin response test: Urine specific gravity increases to 1.035 after 10 hours of water deprivation and the test is stopped.

214. Muscle biopsy—left cranial tibialis muscle: The animal goes into cardiac arrest during induction of anesthesia. Cardiopulmonary resuscitation is unsuccessful.

215. Nerve conduction studies: Conduction velocity is normal in all peripheral nerves tested. There are no clinical signs or test results warranting this procedure in this animal. The dog has a prolonged recovery from anesthesia.

216. Neurologic examination:
Cranial nerves: pupillary light reflexes slow; no other abnormalities
Spinal reflexes:
            Forelimb—withdrawal: normal
            Extensor carpi radialis: normal to hyper
            Hindlimb—withdrawal: normal
            Patellar (quadriceps): normal to hyper
            Perineal: normal
Conscious proprioception: appears reduced in all 4 limbs
Mentation: depressed, possibly disoriented
Cervical pain: evident when neck is flexed or extended
Gait: ataxic; no intention tremors or dysmetria

217. Peripheral nerve biopsy: The animal goes into cardiac arrest during induction of anesthesia. Cardiopulmonary resuscitation is unsuccessful.

218. Survey radiographs—thoracic: An increase in soft-tissue density is observed in the cranial mediastinum, and is pushing the trachea dorsally. A moderate to marked amount of pleural effusion is present, and is obscuring the cardiac silhouette.

219. Survey radiographs—abdominal: mild generalized hepatomegaly

220. Survey radiographs—cervical spine: The dog goes into cardiac arrest during induction of anesthesia. Cardiopulmonary resuscitation is unsuccessful.

221. Survey radiographs—thoracolumbar spine: The dog goes into cardiac arrest during induction of anesthesia. Cardiopulmonary resuscitation is unsuccessful.

222. Survey radiographs—lumbosacral spine: The dog goes into cardiac arrest during induction of anesthesia. Cardiopulmonary resuscitation is unsuccessful.

223. Baseline serum T_4 (thyroxine) concentration: 7 nmol/L [0.5 μg/dl]
(Normal values = 10–50 nmol/L [0.8–3.9 μg/dl])

224. Serum Biochemical Profile

Analyte	Traditional Units	SI Units	Normal Values Traditional Units	Normal Values SI Units
Sodium	148 mEq/L	148 mmol/L	145–158 mEq/L	145–158 mmol/L
Potassium	4.4 mEq/L	4.4 mmol/L	3.6–5.8 mEq/L	3.6–5.8 mmol/L
Chloride	106 mEq/L	106 mmol/L	105–122 mEq/L	105–122 mmol/L
Calcium	10.1 mEq/L	2.51 mmol/L	9.0–11.8 mEq/L	2.24–2.95 mmol/L
Phosphorus	3.87 mEq/L	1.25 mmol/L	1.55–8.05 mEq/L	0.5–2.6 mmol/L
Urea	8.7 mg/dl	3.1 mmol/L	5.9–27.2 mg/dl	2.1–9.7 mmol/L
Creatinine	1.05 mg/dl	93 μmol/L	0.62–1.64 mg/dl	55–145 μmol/L
Glucose	112 mg/dl	6.2 mmol/L	60–158 mg/dl	3.3–8.7 mmol/L
Cholesterol	214 mg/dl	5.53 mmol/L	106–367 mg/dl	2.74–9.5 mmol/L
Total bilirubin	0.12 mg/dl	2 μmol/L	0–0.41 mg/dl	0–7 mmol/L
Amylase	927 IU/L	927 U/L	400–1800 IU/L	400–1800 U/L
ALP	58 IU/L	58 U/L	0–200 IU/L	0–200 U/L
AST	20 IU/L	20 U/L	10–50 IU/L	10–50 U/L
ALT	38 IU/L	38 U/L	0–130 IU/L	0–130 U/L
GGT	3 IU/L	3 U/L	0–6 IU/L	0–6 U/L
Creatine kinase	69 IU/L	69 U/L	0–460 IU/L	0–460 U/L
Total protein	5.8 g/dl	58 g/L	5.0–7.5 g/dl	50–75 g/L
Albumin	3.0 g/dl	30 g/L	2.2–3.5 g/dl	22–35 g/L
Globulins	2.8 g/dl	28 g/L	2.2–4.5 g/dl	22–45 g/L

ALT = alanine aminotransferase; ALP = alkaline phosphatase; AST = aspartate aminotransferase; GGT = γ-glutamyl transpeptidase.

225. Ultrasound—cardiac: no abnormal findings

226. Ultrasound—abdominal: Generalized hepatomegaly is apparent, with no change in hepatic echodensity. Both adrenal glands are visible.

227. Urinalysis

Parameter	Result	Normal Values
Collection method	cystocentesis	
Color/turbidity	yellow/clear	yellow/clear
Specific gravity	1.051	1.001–1.080
pH	6.0	4.5–8.5
Glucose	negative	negative
Ketones	negative	negative
Bilirubin	negative	negative
Occult blood	negative	negative
Protein	negative	negative to trace
RBC/high-power field	0	0–5
WBC/high-power field	0–3	0–5
Casts/low-power field	none	occasional hyaline
Epithelial cells/high-power field	none	occasional
Bacteria/high-power field	none	none
Crystals/high-power field	none	variable

pH = –log hydrogen ion concentration; RBC = red blood cell; WBC = white blood cell.

228. Urine culture: moderate numbers of *Escherichia coli* are cultured.

229. Abdominocentesis:
Appearance: beige, opaque, foul-smelling
Nucleated cell count: $12.0 \times 10^3/\mu l$ ($12 \times 10^9/L$)
Protein: 4.3 g/dl (43 g/L)
Specific gravity: 1.031
Cytologic description: many degenerative neutrophils and bands, some containing rod-shaped bacteria
Shortly after your abdominocentesis the dog becomes more depressed, develops signs of shock, and exhibits abdominal discomfort.

230. Exploratory laparotomy: No abnormal findings. Excessive hemorrhage was evident during and after surgery.

231. Mucosal bleeding time: 2.0 minutes (normal = 1.0–3.2 minutes)

232. Transtracheal wash: No abnormal findings. Aerobic bacterial culture is negative. The procedure exacerbates the cat's dyspnea and it has to be placed in an oxygen cage for several hours before it is stable.

233. Gastroduodenoscopy—examination and biopsy: The proximal duodenal mucosa shows patchy hyperemia. Biopsies reveal marked infiltration of the submucosa and lamina propria with lymphocytes, plasma cells, and a few macrophages. Gastric biopsies are normal.

234. Proctoscopy and colonoscopy—examination and biopsy: Several mucosal erosions and areas of hyperemia are visible. Biopsies show infiltration of the submucosa and lamina propria with lymphocytes, plasma cells, and a few neutrophils.

235. Intestinal biopsy via laparotomy: No abnormal findings. The dog seems to bleed excessively during and after surgery.

236. Splenoportogram: Normal. The dog seems to bleed excessively during and after the procedure.

237. Hepatic biopsy: The animal goes into cardiac arrest during the procedure. Cardiopulmonary resuscitation is unsuccessful.

238. Rhinotomy: No abnormal findings. The dog seems to bleed excessively throughout and after the procedure. A blood transfusion is required.

239. Fundoscopic examination:
Left eye: serous retinal detachment
Right eye: multiple subretinal hemorrhages; white raised subretinal lesions
Interpretation: vasculitis; chorioretinitis and retinal detachment

240. Rocky Mountain spotted fever titer: No detectable titer

241. Survey radiographs—nasal series: No abnormal findings. There are no clinical signs or test results warranting this procedure (which requires general anesthesia) in this patient.

242. Rhinoscopy—examination and biopsy: No abnormal findings. There are no clinical signs or test results warranting this procedure in this patient.

243. Traumatic nasal flush: No abnormal findings. There are no clinical signs or test results warranting this procedure in this patient.

244. Fine-needle aspirate of mass: Aspirate of splenic mass is nondiagnostic.

245. Serum cobalamin: 408 ng/L (normal = 225–660 ng/L)

246. Serum folate: 9.1 µg/L (normal = 6.7–17.4 µg/L)

247. Fat absorption test: The test cannot be performed because the dog is anorexic.

248. Serum osmolality: 332 mOsm/kg (normal = 295–315 mOsm/kg)

249. Urine cortisol:creatinine ratio: 0.1×10^{-6} (normal $< 10 \times 10^{-6}$)

250. Bronchoscopy—examination and sampling: Mild to moderate generalized erythema of the lower airways plus increased mucous accumulation within the airways. Bronchial mucosal biopsies reveal eosinophilic inflammation.

251. Fluoroscopy—thorax: Normal other than microcardia.

252. Fluoroscopy—gastric (in conjunction with upper gastrointestinal [GI] contrast study): Normal, but the dog vomits the contrast media before the study can be completed.

253. Thoracotomy: A nonresectable cranial mediastinal mass is identified during surgery. Biopsy results reveal lymphosarcoma. Postoperatively the cat develops pyothorax caused by a nosocomial infection with *Pseudomonas aeruginosa*, which proves fatal.

254. Pericardiocentesis: You obtain fresh blood because you have punctured the heart and there is no pericardial effusion. The dog goes into cardiac arrest and cannot be resuscitated.

255. Arterial Blood Gas Analysis

Parameter	Result	Normal Values
pH	7.29	7.351–7.463
PCO_2	27 mmHg	30.8–42.8 mmHg
PO_2	89 mmHg	80.9–103.3 mmHg
HCO_3^-	13 mEq/L	18.8–25.6 mEq/L

HCO_3^- = bicarbonate; PCO_2 = partial pressure of carbon dioxide; pH = –log hydrogen ion concentration; PO_2 = partial pressure of oxygen.

256. Cardiac catheterization: The dog goes into cardiac arrest during induction of anesthesia. Cardiopulmonary resuscitation is unsuccessful.

257. Cerebrospinal Fluid Collection and Analysis

Parameter	Result	Normal Values
Protein	0.15 g/L (15 mg/dl)	0.10–0.30 g/L (10–30 mg/dl)
Nucleated cells	0.002×10^9/L	0.0–0.002×10^9/L

Cells are composed primarily of small mononuclear cells.

There are no clinical indications in this patient warranting such an invasive diagnostic procedure. The dog has a prolonged recovery from anesthesia.

258. Computerized tomography—abdomen: Thickening of the caudodorsal bladder wall is revealed. Although this is a means of identifying bladder lesions, there are less expensive methods.

259. Contrast radiographs—myelogram: Normal. The dog has a prolonged recovery from anesthesia. There are no clinical indications warranting such an invasive diagnostic procedure in this animal.

260. Contrast radiographs—cystogram: Radiodense calculi in the bladder. (These were seen on survey radiographs and so this procedure, which requires anesthesia, gives no added information concerning this patient.) The dog has a prolonged recovery from anesthesia.

261. Contrast radiographs—upper gastrointestinal study: The gastrointestinal tract appears normal, but the intestinal loops are displaced cranially and dorsally by a large, fluid-filled structure in the mid-caudal abdomen.

262. Water deprivation/vasopressin response test: Starting urine specific gravity was 1.011. After 16 hours of water deprivation, the dog was 5% dehydrated. Urine specific gravity at that time was 1.017. Vasopressin is administered and the urine specific gravity increases to 1.020.

263. Muscle biopsy—left cranial tibialis muscle: No abnormal findings. There are no clinical signs or test results warranting such an invasive diagnostic procedure in this animal. The dog has a prolonged recovery from anesthesia.

264. Neurologic examination: No abnormal findings other than weakness. Postural reactions cannot be evaluated because of the dog's size and profound weakness.

265. Peripheral nerve biopsy—right distal peroneal nerve: No abnormal findings. There are no clinical indications warranting such an invasive diagnostic test in this animal. The dog has a prolonged recovery from anesthesia.

266. Survey radiographs—thoracic: mild bronchial pattern with an interstitial component

267. Survey radiographs—abdominal: poor abdominal detail because the dog is thin; fluid-filled bowel loops are also seen.

268. Survey radiographs—cervical spine: No abnormal findings. There are no clinical signs or test results warranting this procedure (which requires general anesthesia) in this patient. The dog has a prolonged recovery from anesthesia.

269. Survey radiographs—thoracolumbar spine: No abnormal findings. There are no clinical signs or test results warranting this procedure (which requires general anesthesia) in this patient. The dog has a prolonged recovery from anesthesia.

270. Survey radiographs—lumbosacral spine: No abnormal findings. There are no clinical signs or test results warranting this procedure (which requires general anesthesia) in this patient. The dog has a prolonged recovery from anesthesia.

271. Baseline serum T_4 (thyroxine) concentration: 14 nmol/L (1.1 μg/dl)
Normal values = 12–50 nmol/L (0.9–3.9 μg/dl)

272. Serum Biochemical Profile

Analyte	Traditional Units	SI Units	Normal Values Traditional Units	Normal Values SI Units
Sodium	153 mEq/L	153 mmol/L	150–165 mEq/L	150–165 mmol/L
Potassium	5.0 mEq/L	5.0 mmol/L	3.7–5.8 mEq/L	3.7–5.8 mmol/L
Chloride	116 mEq/L	116 mmol/L	112–129 mEq/L	112–129 mmol/L
Calcium	11.4 mEq/L	2.85 mmol/L	8.9–11.6 mEq/L	2.23–2.9 mmol/L
Phosphorus	5.6 mEq/L	1.81 mmol/L	3.2–8.7 mEq/L	1.03–2.82 mmol/L
Urea	21.8 mg/dl	7.8 mmol/L	14–28 mg/dl	5–10 mmol/L
Creatinine	1.3 mg/dl	117 μmol/L	0.84–2.04 mg/dl	75–180 μmol/L
Glucose	128 mg/dl	7.1 mmol/L	63–162 mg/dl	3.5–9.0 mmol/L
Cholesterol	112 mg/dl	2.89 mmol/L	58–232 mg/dl	1.5–6.0 mmol/L
Total bilirubin	0 mg/dl	0 μmol/L	0–0.23 mg/dl	0–4 mmol/L
Amylase	967 IU/L	967 U/L	700–2000 IU/L	700–2000 U/L
ALP	32 IU/L	32 U/L	0–90 IU/L	0–90 U/L
AST	33 IU/L	33 U/L	10–59 IU/L	10–59 U/L
ALT	29 IU/L	29 U/L	10–75 IU/L	10–75 U/L
GGT	0 IU/L	0 U/L	0–2 IU/L	0–2 U/L
Creatine kinase	310 IU/L	310 U/L	0–580 IU/L	0–580 U/L
Total protein	8.1 g/dl	81 g/L	6.0–8.2 g/dl	60–82 g/L
Albumin	3.8 g/dl	38 g/L	2.5–3.9 g/dl	25–39 g/L
Globulins	4.3 g/dl	43 g/L	2.6–5.0 g/dl	26–50 g/L

ALT = alanine aminotransferase; ALP = alkaline phosphatase; AST = aspartate aminotransferase; GGT = γ-glutamyl transpeptidase.

273. Ultrasound—cardiac: No abnormal cardiac findings. A large, soft-tissue mass is visualized cranial to the heart.

274. Ultrasound—abdominal: Small to moderate amount of fluid in the urinary bladder. The caudodorsal bladder wall seems to be thickened and irregular, but the bladder is not distended enough to confirm this.

275. Urinalysis

Parameter	Result	Normal Values
Collection method	cystocentesis	
Color/turbidity	yellow/clear	yellow/clear
Specific gravity	1.021	1.001–1.065
pH	6.0	4.5–8.5
Glucose	negative	negative
Ketones	negative	negative
Bilirubin	trace	trace to 1+
Occult blood	negative	negative
Protein	negative	negative to trace
RBC/high-power field	0–2	0–5
WBC/high-power field	0–3	0–5
Casts/low-power field	none	occasional hyaline
Epithelial cells/high-power field	none	occasional
Bacteria/high-power field	none	none
Crystals/high-power field	few phosphate	variable

pH = −log hydrogen ion concentration; RBC = red blood cell; WBC = white blood cell.

276. Exploratory laparotomy: no abnormal findings

277. Transtracheal wash: The sample is markedly cellular, comprised primarily of eosinophils with a small number of neutrophils and mononuclear cells; aerobic bacterial culture is negative.

278. Gastroduodenoscopy—examination and biopsy: No abnormal findings. The dog has a prolonged recovery from anesthesia.

279. Intestinal biopsy via laparotomy: Full thickness biopsies show infiltration of the submucosa and lamina propria with lymphocytes, plasma cells, and a few macrophages.

280. Splenoportogram: An extrahepatic portosystemic shunt is identified.

281. Hepatic biopsy: vacuolization of hepatocytes observed; most consistent with steroid hepatopathy

282. Rhinotomy: No abnormal findings. There are no clinical signs or test results warranting this invasive procedure in this patient. The dog has a prolonged recovery from anesthesia.

283. Survey radiographs—nasal series: No abnormal findings. There are no clinical signs or test results warranting this procedure (which requires general anesthesia) in this patient. The dog has a prolonged recovery from anesthesia.

284. Rhinoscopy—examination and biopsy: No abnormal findings. There are no clinical signs or test results warranting this invasive procedure in this patient. The dog has a prolonged recovery from anesthesia.

285. Traumatic nasal flush: No abnormal findings. There are no clinical signs or test results warranting this procedure in this patient. The dog has a prolonged recovery from anesthesia.

286. Fine-needle aspirate of mass: A percutaneous aspirate of the suspected bladder mass is not possible.

287. Bronchoscopy—examination and sampling: Normal. The dog has a prolonged recovery from anesthesia.

288. Thoracotomy: No abnormalities are identified. The dog chews off its chest tube postoperatively and dies of acute pnemothorax.

289. Complete Blood Count

Parameter	Traditional Units	SI Units	Normal Values Traditional Units	Normal Values SI Units
Hemoglobin	15 g/dl	150 g/L	13.2–19.2 g/dl	132–193 g/L
Hematocrit	42.5%	0.425 L/L	38–57%	0.38–0.57 L/L
Erythrocytes	6.7×10^6/L	6.7×10^{12}/L	$5.6–8.5 \times 10^6$/μl	$5.6–8.5 \times 10^{12}$/L
MCV	63.5 mm^3	63.5 fl	62–71 mm^3	62–71 fl
MCH	22.4 pg	22.4 pg	22–25 pg	22–25 pg
MCHC	35.3%	353 g/L	33.7–36.5%	337–365 g/L
Reticulocytes	0%	0%	0–1.5%	0–1.5%
Platelets	350×10^3/μl	350×10^9/L	$145–440 \times 10^3$/μl	$145–440 \times 10^9$/L
Total nucleated cell count	11.05×10^3/μl	11.05×10^9/L	$6.1–17.4 \times 10^3$/μl	$6.1–17.4 \times 10^9$/L
Neutrophils	6.3×10^3/μl (57%)	6.3×10^9/L (59%)	$3.9–12 \times 10^3$/μl	$3.9–12 \times 10^9$/L
Band neutrophils	0	0	$0–1.0 \times 10^3$/μl	$0–1.0 \times 10^9$/μl
Lymphocytes	1.5×10^3/μl (13.6%)	1.5×10^9/L (14%)	$0.8–3.6 \times 10^3$/μl	$0.8–3.6 \times 10^9$/L
Monocytes	0.75×10^3/μl (6.8%)	0.75×10^9/L (7%)	$0–1.8 \times 10^3$/μl	$0–1.8 \times 10^9$/L
Eosinophils	2.2×10^3/μl (20%)	2.2×10^9/L (16%)	$0–1.9 \times 10^3$/μl	$0–1.9 \times 10^9$/L
Basophils	0.3×10^3/μl (2.6%)	0.3×10^9/L (3%)	$0–0.2 \times 10^3$/μl	$0–0.2 \times 10^9$/L

MCH = mean corpuscular hemoglobin; MCHC = mean corpuscular hemoglobin concentration; MCV = mean corpuscular volume.

290. Computerized tomography—abdomen: Thickened bowel walls; although this is a means of identifying some intestinal lesions, there are less expensive methods.

291. Water deprivation/vasopressin response test: The shock and bradycardia worsen and the dog goes into cardiac arrest after 2 hours.

292. Survey radiographs—abdominal: Poor abdominal detail because the dog is thin; microhepatica; small, radiodense objects in the urinary bladder.

293. Serum Biochemical Profile

Analyte	Traditional Units	SI Units	Normal Values Traditional Units	Normal Values SI Units
Sodium	153 mEq/L	153 mmol/L	145–158 mEq/L	145–158 mmol/L
Potassium	4.7 mEq/L	4.7 mmol/L	3.6–5.8 mEq/L	3.6–5.8 mmol/L
Chloride	113 mEq/L	113 mmol/L	105–122 mEq/L	105–122 mmol/L
Calcium	10.2 mEq/L	2.54 mmol/L	9.0–11.8 mEq/L	2.24–2.95 mmol/L
Phosphorus	5.57 mEq/L	1.8 mmol/L	1.55–8.05 mEq/L	0.5–2.6 mmol/L
Urea	16 mg/dl	5.7 mmol/L	5.9–27.2 mg/dl	2.1–9.7 mmol/L
Creatinine	1.4 mg/dl	125 µmol/L	0.62–1.64 mg/dl	55–145 µmol/L
Glucose	112 mg/dl	6.2 mmol/L	60–158 mg/dl	3.3–8.7 mmol/L
Cholesterol	186 mg/dl	4.79 mmol/L	106–367 mg/dl	2.74–9.5 mmol/L
Total bilirubin	0.18 mg/dl	3 µmol/L	0–0.41 mg/dl	0–7 mmol/L
Amylase	651 IU/L	651 U/L	400–1800 IU/L	400–1800 U/L
ALP	76 IU/L	76 U/L	0–200 IU/L	0–200 U/L
AST	16 IU/L	16 U/L	10–50 IU/L	10–50 U/L
ALT	49 IU/L	49 U/L	0–130 IU/L	0–130 U/L
GGT	2 IU/L	2 U/L	0–6 IU/L	0–6 U/L
Creatine kinase	154 IU/L	154 U/L	0–460 IU/L	0–460 U/L
Total protein	6.7 g/dl	67 g/L	5.0–7.5 g/dl	50–75 g/L
Albumin	3.1 g/dl	31 g/L	2.2–3.5 g/dl	22–35 g/L
Globulins	3.6 g/dl	36 g/L	2.2–4.5 g/dl	22–45 g/L

ALT = alanine aminotransferase; ALP = alkaline phosphatase; AST = aspartate aminotransferase; GGT = γ-glutamyl transpeptidase.

294. Ultrasound—cardiac: bradycardia; decreased chamber size with normal wall thickness

295. Ultrasound—abdominal: thickened small intestinal walls

296. Urinalysis

Parameter	Result	Normal Values
Collection method	cystocentesis	
Color/turbidity	yellow/clear	yellow/clear
Specific gravity	1.048	1.001–1.065
pH	6.0	4.5–8.5
Glucose	negative	negative
Ketones	negative	negative
Bilirubin	trace	trace to 1+
Occult blood	negative	negative
Protein	negative	negative to trace
RBC/high-power field	0–2	0–5
WBC/high-power field	0–3	0–5
Casts/low-power field	none	occasional hyaline
Epithelial cells/high-power field	none	occasional
Bacteria/high-power field	none	none
Crystals/high-power field	few phosphate	variable

pH = –log hydrogen ion concentration; RBC = red blood cell; WBC = white blood cell.

297. Exploratory laparotomy: Bilateral adrenal enlargement and mild generalized hepatomegaly. This procedure is very inappropriate for this patient because other noninvasive diagnostic tests can establish the diagnosis.

298. Transtracheal wash: The procedure is stopped because the bradycardia and shock become worse.

299. Hepatic biopsy: hepatic atrophy and lobular collapse.

300. Bronchoscopy—examination and sampling: normal. The lethargy and vomiting become worse.

301. Thoracotomy: No abnormalities are identified. The dog never recovers from general anesthesia, lapses into a coma, and dies.

302. Complete Blood Count

Parameter	Traditional Units	SI Units	Normal Values Traditional Units	Normal Values SI Units
Hemoglobin	17 g/dl	170 g/L	13.2–19.2 g/dl	132–193 g/L
Hematocrit	40.8%	0.408 L/L	38–57%	0.38–0.57 L/L
Erythrocytes	$6.01 \times 10^6/\mu l$	$6.01 \times 10^{12}/L$	$5.6–8.5 \times 10^6/\mu l$	$5.6–8.5 \times 10^{12}/L$
MCV	67.9 mm^3	67.9 fl	62–71 mm^3	62–71 fl
MCH	25 pg	25 pg	22–25 pg	22–25 pg
MCHC	365%	365 g/L	33.7–36.5%	337–365 g/L
Reticulocytes	0%	0%	0–1.5%	0–1.5%
Platelets	$322 \times 10^3/\mu l$	$322 \times 10^9/L$	$145–440 \times 10^3/\mu l$	$145–440 \times 10^9/L$
Total nucleated cell count	$17 \times 10^3/\mu l$	$17 \times 10^9/L$	$6.1–17.4 \times 10^3/\mu l$	$6.1–17.4 \times 10^9/L$
Neutrophils	$15.0 \times 10^3/\mu l$ (88%)	$15.0 \times 10^9/L$ (88%)	$3.9–12 \times 10^3/\mu l$	$3.9–12 \times 10^9/L$
Band neutrophils	$0.2 \times 10^3/\mu l$ (1%)	$0.2 \times 10^3/L$ (1%)	$0–1.0 \times 10^3/\mu l$	$0–1.0 \times 10^9/L$
Lymphocytes	$0.85 \times 10^3/\mu l$ (5%)	$0.85 \times 10^9/L$ (5%)	$0.8–3.6 \times 10^3/\mu l$	$0.8–3.6 \times 10^9/L$
Monocytes	$0.85 \times 10^3/\mu l$ (5%)	$0.85 \times 10^9/L$ (5%)	$0–1.8 \times 10^3/\mu l$	$0–1.8 \times 10^9/L$
Eosinophils	$0.2 \times 10^3/\mu l$ (1%)	$0.2 \times 10^9/L$ (1%)	$0–1.9 \times 10^3/\mu l$	$0–1.9 \times 10^9/L$
Basophils	0	0	$0–0.2 \times 10^3/\mu l$	$0–0.2 \times 10^9/L$

MCH = mean corpuscular hemoglobin; MCHC = mean corpuscular hemoglobin concentration; MCV = mean corpuscular volume.

303. Computerized tomography—abdomen: The dog goes into cardiac arrest during induction of anesthesia. Cardiopulmonary resuscitation is unsuccessful.

304. Water deprivation/vasopressin response test: Starting urine specific gravity was 1.020. After 12 hours of water deprivation, the urine specific gravity increases to 1.030. The test is discontinued at that time.

305. Survey radiographs—abdominal: A large, tubular structure is seen in the mid-caudal abdomen. Intestinal loops are displaced dorsally and cranially.

306. Serum Biochemical Profile

Analyte	Traditional Units	SI Units	Normal Values Traditional Units	Normal Values SI Units
Sodium	147 mEq/L	147 mmol/L	145–158 mEq/L	145–158 mmol/L
Potassium	5.0 mEq/L	5.0 mmol/L	3.6–5.8 mEq/L	3.6–5.8 mmol/L
Chloride	110 mEq/L	110 mmol/L	105–122 mEq/L	105–122 mmol/L
Calcium	9.3 mEq/L	2.32 mmol/L	9.0–11.8 mEq/L	2.24–2.95 mmol/L
Phosphorus	6.5 mEq/L	2.1 mmol/L	1.55–8.05 mEq/L	0.5–2.6 mmol/L
Urea	23 mg/dl	8.2 mmol/L	5.9–27.2 mg/dl	2.1–9.7 mmol/L
Creatinine	1.1 mg/dl	95 μmol/L	0.62–1.64 mg/dl	55–145 μmol/L
Glucose	106 mg/dl	5.9 mmol/L	60–158 mg/dl	3.3–8.7 mmol/L
Cholesterol	132 mg/dl	3.4 mmol/L	106–367 mg/dl	2.74–9.5 mmol/L
Total bilirubin	0.18 mg/dl	3 μmol/L	0–0.41 mg/dl	0–7 mmol/L
Amylase	922 IU/L	922 U/L	400–1800 IU/L	400–1800 U/L
ALP	75 IU/L	75 U/L	0–200 IU/L	0–200 U/L
AST	42 IU/L	42 U/L	10–50 IU/L	10–50 U/L
ALT	63 IU/L	63 U/L	0–130 IU/L	0–130 U/L
GGT	4 IU/L	4 U/L	0–6 IU/L	0–6 U/L
Creatine kinase	237 IU/L	237 U/L	0–460 IU/L	0–460 U/L
Total protein	7.1 g/dl	71 g/L	5.0–7.5 g/dl	50–75 g/L
Albumin	2.8 g/dl	28 g/L	2.2–3.5 g/dl	22–35 g/L
Globulins	4.3 g/dl	43 g/L	2.2–4.5 g/dl	22–45 g/L

ALT = alanine aminotransferase; ALP = alkaline phosphatase; AST = aspartate aminotransferase; GGT = γ-glutamyl transpeptidase.

307. Ultrasound—abdominal: microhepatica; few hepatic vessels visible; calculi in bladder

308. Urinalysis

Parameter	Result	Normal Values
Collection method	cystocentesis	
Color/turbidity	yellow/clear	yellow/clear
Specific gravity	1.013	1.001–1.065
pH	6.0	4.5–8.5
Glucose	negative	negative
Ketones	negative	negative
Bilirubin	trace	trace to 1+
Occult blood	trace	negative
Protein	negative	negative to trace
RBC/high-power field	5–10	0–5
WBC/high-power field	5–10	0–5
Casts/low-power field	none	occasional hyaline
Epithelial cells/high-power field	none	occasional
Bacteria/high-power field	trace	none
Crystals/high-power field	few phosphate	variable

pH = −log hydrogen ion concentration; RBC = red blood cell; WBC = white blood cell.

309. Exploratory laparotomy: Palpation of the bladder reveals thickening of the caudo-dorsal bladder wall. A cystotomy performed to visualize the area shows an irregular friable mass extending from the trigone area into the bladder lumen. If this procedure is performed on the first day of your diagnostic testing, it probably was not preceded by logical diagnostic testing.

310. Thoracotomy: Normal. Postoperatively the dog goes into cardiac arrest and cannot be resuscitated.

311. Complete Blood Count

Parameter	Traditional Units	SI Units	Normal Values Traditional Units	Normal Values SI Units
Hemoglobin	15 g/dl	150 g/L	13.2–19.2 g/dl	132–193 g/L
Hematocrit	40.8%	0.408 L/L	38–57%	0.38–0.57 L/L
Erythrocytes	$6.01 \times 10^6/\mu l$	$6.01 \times 10^{12}/L$	$5.6–8.5 \times 10^6/\mu l$	$5.6–8.5 \times 10^{12}/L$
MCV	67.9 mm³	67.9 fl	62–71 mm³	62–71 fl
MCH	25 pg	25 pg	22–25 pg	22–25 pg
MCHC	36.5%	365 g/L	33.7–36.5%	337–365 g/L
Reticulocytes	0%	0%	0–1.5%	0–1.5%
Platelets	$322 \times 10^3/\mu l$	$322 \times 10^9/L$	$145–440 \times 10^3/\mu l$	$145–440 \times 10^9/L$
Total nucleated cell count	$14.5 \times 10^3/\mu l$	$14.5 \times 10^9/L$	$6.1–17.4 \times 10^3/\mu l$	$6.1–17.4 \times 10^9/L$
Neutrophils	$10.4 \times 10^3/\mu l$ (72%)	$10.4 \times 10^9/L$ (72%)	$3.9–12 \times 10^3/\mu l$	$3.9–12 \times 10^9/L$
Band neutrophils	$0.3 \times 10^3/\mu l$ (2%)	$0.3 \times 10^3/L$ (2%)	$0–1.0 \times 10^3/\mu l$	$0–1.0 \times 10^9/L$
Lymphocytes	$1.5 \times 10^3/\mu l$ (10%)	$1.5 \times 10^9/L$ (10%)	$0.8–3.6 \times 10^3/\mu l$	$0.8–3.6 \times 10^9/L$
Monocytes	$1.7 \times 10^3/\mu l$ (12%)	$1.7 \times 10^9/L$ (12%)	$0–1.8 \times 10^3/\mu l$	$0–1.8 \times 10^9/L$
Eosinophils	$0.6 \times 10^3/\mu l$ (4%)	$0.6 \times 10^9/L$ (4%)	$0–1.9 \times 10^3/\mu l$	$0–1.9 \times 10^9/L$
Basophils	0	0	$0–0.2 \times 10^3/\mu l$	$0–0.2 \times 10^9/L$

MCH = mean corpuscular hemoglobin; MCHC = mean corpuscular hemoglobin concentration; MCV = mean corpuscular volume.

312. Computerized tomography—abdomen: microhepatica and decreased hepatic vessel number and size.

313. Water deprivation/vasopressin response test: Starting urine specific gravity was 1.015. After 4 hours of water deprivation, the dog's vomiting becomes worse and she is mildly azotemic. The test is discontinued.

314. Serum Biochemical Profile

Analyte	Traditional Units	SI Units	Normal Values Traditional Units	Normal Values SI Units
Sodium	142 mEq/L	142 mmol/L	145–158 mEq/L	145–158 mmol/L
Potassium	4.6 mEq/L	4.6 mmol/L	3.6–5.8 mEq/L	3.6–5.8 mmol/L
Chloride	114 mEq/L	114 mmol/L	105–122 mEq/L	105–122 mmol/L
Calcium	9.2 mEq/L	2.29 mmol/L	9.0–11.8 mEq/L	2.24–2.95 mmol/L
Phosphorus	5.7 mEq/L	1.84 mmol/L	1.55–8.05 mEq/L	0.5–2.6 mmol/L
Urea	9 mg/dl	3.2 mmol/L	5.9–27.2 mg/dl	2.1–9.7 mmol/L
Creatinine	0.7 mg/dl	62 μmol/L	0.62–1.64 mg/dl	55–145 μmol/L
Glucose	93 mg/dl	5.2 mmol/L	60–158 mg/dl	3.3–8.7 mmol/L
Cholesterol	227 mg/dl	5.9 mmol/L	106–367 mg/dl	2.74–9.5 mmol/L
Total bilirubin	0.18 mg/dl	3 μmol/L	0–0.41 mg/dl	0–7 mmol/L
Amylase	922 IU/L	922 U/L	400–1800 IU/L	400–1800 U/L
ALP	134 IU/L	134 U/L	0–200 IU/L	0–200 U/L
AST	42 IU/L	42 U/L	10–50 IU/L	10–50 U/L
ALT	63 IU/L	63 U/L	0–130 IU/L	0–130 U/L
GGT	4 IU/L	4 U/L	0–6 IU/L	0–6 U/L
Creatine kinase	237 IU/L	237 U/L	0–460 IU/L	0–460 U/L
Total protein	4.1 g/dl	41 g/L	5.0–7.5 g/dl	50–75 g/L
Albumin	2.0 g/dl	20 g/L	2.2–3.5 g/dl	22–35 g/L
Globulins	2.1 g/dl	21 g/L	2.2–4.5 g/dl	22–45 g/L

ALT = alanine aminotransferase; ALP = alkaline phosphatase; AST = aspartate aminotransferase; GGT = γ-glutamyl transpeptidase.

315. Ultrasound—abdominal: large, fluid-filled uterus

316. Urinalysis

Parameter	Result	Normal Values
Collection method	free flow	
Color/turbidity	red-tinged/clear	yellow/clear
Specific gravity	1.035	1.001–1.065
pH	6.0	4.5–8.5
Glucose	negative	negative
Ketones	negative	negative
Bilirubin	1+	trace to 1+
Occult blood	2+	negative
Protein	1+	negative to trace
RBC/high-power field	50+	0–5
WBC/high-power field	2–5	0–5
Casts/low-power field	none	occasional hyaline
Epithelial cells/high-power field	3–5 squamous epithelial cells	occasional
Bacteria/high-power field	none	none
Crystals/high-power field	none	variable

pH = –log hydrogen ion concentration; RBC = red blood cell; WBC = white blood cell.

317. Exploratory laparotomy: The duodenal and proximal jejunal walls are thickened.

318. Thoracotomy: The owners take the dog to another clinic for a second opinion and find that there is no indication for a thoracotomy. They file a complaint with the local veterinary medical association.

319. Complete Blood Count

Parameter	Traditional Units	SI Units	Normal Values Traditional Units	Normal Values SI Units
Hemoglobin	14.2 g/dl	142 g/L	13.2–19.2 g/dl	132–193 g/L
Hematocrit	40.0%	0.400 L/L	38–57%	0.38–0.57 L/L
Erythrocytes	$6.1 \times 10^6/\mu l$	$6.1 \times 10^{12}/L$	$5.6–8.5 \times 10^6/\mu l$	$5.6–8.5 \times 10^{12}/L$
MCV	67 mm³	67 fl	62–71 mm³	62–71 fl
MCH	24 pg	24 pg	22–25 pg	22–25 pg
MCHC	36%	360 g/L	33.7–36.5%	337–365 g/L
Reticulocytes	0%	0%	0–1.5%	0–1.5%
Platelets	$322 \times 10^3/\mu l$	$322 \times 10^9/L$	$145–440 \times 10^3/\mu l$	$145–440 \times 10^9/L$
Total nucleated cell count	$29.7 \times 10^3/\mu l$	$29.7 \times 10^9/L$	$6.1–17.4 \times 10^3/\mu l$	$6.1–17.4 \times 10^9/L$
Neutrophils	$27.0 \times 10^3/\mu l$ (91%)	$27.0 \times 10^9/L$ (91%)	$3.9–12 \times 10^3/\mu l$	$3.9–12 \times 10^9/L$
Band neutrophils	$1.2 \times 10^3/\mu l$ (4%)	$1.2 \times 10^3/L$ (4%)	$0–1.0 \times 10^3/\mu l$	$0–1.0 \times 10^9/L$
Lymphocytes	$0.9 \times 10^3/\mu l$ (3%)	$0.9 \times 10^9/L$ (3%)	$0.8–3.6 \times 10^3/\mu l$	$0.8–3.6 \times 10^9/L$
Monocytes	$0.6 \times 10^3/\mu l$ (2%)	$0.6 \times 10^9/L$ (2%)	$0–1.8 \times 10^3/\mu l$	$0–1.8 \times 10^9/L$
Eosinophils	0	0	$0–1.9 \times 10^3/\mu l$	$0–1.9 \times 10^9/L$
Basophils	0	0	$0–0.2 \times 10^3/\mu l$	$0–0.2 \times 10^9/L$

MCH = mean corpuscular hemoglobin; MCHC = mean corpuscular hemoglobin concentration; MCV = mean corpuscular volume.

320. Computerized tomography—abdomen: large, fluid-filled uterus.

321. Serum Biochemical Profile

Analyte	Traditional Units	SI Units	Normal Values Traditional Units	Normal Values SI Units
Sodium	147 mEq/L	147 mmol/L	145–158 mEq/L	145–158 mmol/L
Potassium	4.5 mEq/L	4.5 mmol/L	3.6–5.8 mEq/L	3.6–5.8 mmol/L
Chloride	110 mEq/L	110 mmol/L	105–122 mEq/L	105–122 mmol/L
Calcium	9.3 mEq/L	2.32 mmol/L	9.0–11.8 mEq/L	2.24–2.95 mmol/L
Phosphorus	6.5 mEq/L	2.1 mmol/L	1.55–8.05 mEq/L	0.5–2.6 mmol/L
Urea	23 mg/dl	8.2 mmol/L	5.9–27.2 mg/dl	2.1–9.7 mmol/L
Creatinine	1.1 mg/dl	95 μmol/L	0.62–1.64 mg/dl	55–145 μmol/L
Glucose	113 mg/dl	6.3 mmol/L	60–158 mg/dl	3.3–8.7 mmol/L
Cholesterol	278 mg/dl	7.2 mmol/L	106–367 mg/dl	2.74–9.5 mmol/L
Total bilirubin	0.18 mg/dl	3 μmol/L	0–0.41 mg/dl	0–7 mmol/L
Amylase	922 IU/L	922 U/L	400–1800 IU/L	400–1800 U/L
ALP	839 IU/L	839 U/L	0–200 IU/L	0–200 U/L
AST	42 IU/L	42 U/L	10–50 IU/L	10–50 U/L
ALT	63 IU/L	63 U/L	0–130 IU/L	0–130 U/L
GGT	4 IU/L	4 U/L	0–6 IU/L	0–6 U/L
Creatine kinase	237 IU/L	237 U/L	0–460 IU/L	0–460 U/L
Total protein	7.1 g/dl	71 g/L	5.0–7.5 g/dl	50–75 g/L
Albumin	2.8 g/dl	28 g/L	2.2–3.5 g/dl	22–35 g/L
Globulins	4.3 g/dl	43 g/L	2.2–4.5 g/dl	22–45 g/L

ALT = alanine aminotransferase; ALP = alkaline phosphatase; AST = aspartate aminotransferase; GGT = γ-glutamyl transpeptidase.

322. Urinalysis

Parameter	Result	Normal Values
Collection method	free flow	
Color/turbidity	yellow/clear	yellow/clear
Specific gravity	1.035	1.001–1.065
pH	6.5	4.5–8.5
Glucose	negative	negative
Ketones	negative	negative
Bilirubin	trace	trace to 1+
Occult blood	negative	negative
Protein	negative	negative to trace
RBC/high-power field	0–2	0–5
WBC/high-power field	0–3	0–5
Casts/low-power field	none	occasional hyaline
Epithelial cells/high-power field	none	occasional
Bacteria/high-power field	none	none
Crystals/high-power field	none	variable

pH = –log hydrogen ion concentration; RBC = red blood cell; WBC = white blood cell.

323. Exploratory laparotomy: The liver is very small.

324. Complete Blood Count

Parameter	Traditional Units	SI Units	Normal Values Traditional Units	Normal Values SI Units
Hemoglobin	16.8 g/dl	168 g/L	13.2–19.2 g/dl	132–193 g/L
Hematocrit	48%	0.48 L/L	38–57%	0.38–0.57 L/L
Erythrocytes	$7.8 \times 10^6/\mu l$	$7.8 \times 10^{12}/L$	5.6–$8.5 \times 10^6/\mu l$	5.6–$8.5 \times 10^{12}/L$
MCV	62 mm^3	62 fl	62–71 mm^3	62–71 fl
MCH	23.5 pg	23.5 pg	22–25 pg	22–25 pg
MCHC	35%	350 g/L	33.7–36.5%	337–365 g/L
Reticulocytes	0%	0%	0–1.5%	0–1.5%
Platelets	$322 \times 10^3/\mu l$	$322 \times 10^9/L$	145–$440 \times 10^3/\mu l$	145–$440 \times 10^9/L$
Total nucleated cell count	$12.4 \times 10^3/\mu l$	$12.4 \times 10^9/L$	6.1–$17.4 \times 10^3/\mu l$	6.1–$17.4 \times 10^9/L$
Neutrophils	$11.2 \times 10^3/\mu l$ (90%)	$12.2 \times 10^9/L$ (90%)	3.9–$12 \times 10^3/\mu l$	3.9–$12 \times 10^9/L$
Band neutrophils	$0.12 \times 10^3/\mu l$ (1%)	$0.12 \times 10^3/L$ (1%)	0–$1.0 \times 10^3/\mu l$	0–$1.0 \times 10^9/L$
Lymphocytes	$0.9 \times 10^3/\mu l$ (7%)	$0.9 \times 10^9/L$ (7%)	0.8–$3.6 \times 10^3/\mu l$	0.8–$3.6 \times 10^9/L$
Monocytes	$0.2 \times 10^3/\mu l$ (2%)	$0.2 \times 10^9/L$ (2%)	0–$1.8 \times 10^3/\mu l$	0–$1.8 \times 10^9/L$
Eosinophils	0	0	0–$1.9 \times 10^3/\mu l$	0–$1.9 \times 10^9/L$
Basophils	0	0	0–$0.2 \times 10^3/\mu l$	0–$0.2 \times 10^9/L$

MCH = mean corpuscular hemoglobin; MCHC = mean corpuscular hemoglobin concentration; MCV = mean corpuscular volume.

325. Serum Biochemical Profile

Analyte	Traditional Units	SI Units	Normal Values Traditional Units	Normal Values SI Units
Sodium	147 mEq/L	147 mmol/L	145–158 mEq/L	145–158 mmol/L
Potassium	5.0 mEq/L	5.0 mmol/L	3.6–5.8 mEq/L	3.6–5.8 mmol/L
Chloride	110 mEq/L	110 mmol/L	105–122 mEq/L	105–122 mmol/L
Calcium	9.3 mEq/L	2.32 mmol/L	9.0–11.8 mEq/L	2.24–2.95 mmol/L
Phosphorus	6.5 mEq/L	2.1 mmol/L	1.55–8.05 mEq/L	0.5–2.6 mmol/L
Urea	23 mg/dl	8.2 mmol/L	5.9–27.2 mg/dl	2.1–9.7 mmol/L
Creatinine	1.1 mg/dl	95 μmol/L	0.62–1.64 mg/dl	55–145 μmol/L
Glucose	62 mg/dl	3.4 mmol/L	60–158 mg/dl	3.3–8.7 mmol/L
Cholesterol	111 mg/dl	2.9 mmol/L	106–367 mg/dl	2.74–9.5 mmol/L
Total bilirubin	0.18 mg/dl	3 μmol/L	0–0.41 mg/dl	0–7 mmol/L
Amylase	922 IU/L	922 U/L	400–1800 IU/L	400–1800 U/L
ALP	75 IU/L	75 U/L	0–200 IU/L	0–200 U/L
AST	42 IU/L	42 U/L	10–50 IU/L	10–50 U/L
ALT	63 IU/L	63 U/L	0–130 IU/L	0–130 U/L
GGT	4 IU/L	4 U/L	0–6 IU/L	0–6 U/L
Creatine kinase	237 IU/L	237 U/L	0–460 IU/L	0–460 U/L
Total protein	5.7 g/dl	57 g/L	5.0–7.5 g/dl	50–75 g/L
Albumin	2.2 g/dl	22 g/L	2.2–3.5 g/dl	22–35 g/L
Globulins	3.5 g/dl	35 g/L	2.2–4.5 g/dl	22–45 g/L

ALT = alanine aminotransferase; ALP = alkaline phosphatase; AST = aspartate aminotransferase; GGT = γ-glutamyl transpeptidase.

326. Adrenocorticotropic hormone (ACTH) concentration (endogenous): 13 pmol/L [59 pg/ml] (normal = 1–20 pmol/L [4.5–91 pg/ml])

327. Urine protein:creatinine ratio: 0.8 (normal < 1.0)

328. Cardiac catheterization: Normal. There are no clinical signs or test results warranting this invasive procedure in this patient. The dog has a prolonged recovery from anesthesia.

329. Duodenal aspirate culture: 6×10^4 microorganisms/ml (normal < 10^5 microorganisms/ml)

330. Gastroduodenoscopy—examination and biopsy: No abnormal findings. The lethargy and vomiting become worse.

331. Contrast radiographs—cystogram: No abnormal findings in the bladder, but a large, tubular, fluid-density structure is evident in the mid-caudal abdomen.

332. Contrast radiographs—intravenous pyelogram: No abnormal findings in the kidneys or ureters, but a large, tubular, fluid-density structure is evident in the mid-caudal abdomen.

333. Contrast radiographs—splenoportogram: No abnormal vasculature structure is found, but a large, tubular, fluid-density structure is evident in the mid-caudal abdomen.

334. Contrast radiographs—upper gastrointestinal (GI) study: The dog vomits the contrast media, so the study is stopped. However, a large, tubular, fluid-density structure is evident in the mid-caudal abdomen.

335. Intestinal biopsy via laparotomy: No abnormal findings. However, a large, hyperemic, fluid-filled uterus is evident.

Part F
Diagnosis List

PART
F

Directions: Select your diagnosis/diagnoses from the following list of choices. When you are finished, go to Part G.

Acromegaly
Acute polyradiculoneuritis
Adenocarcinoma—intestinal
Allergic bronchitis
Anemia
Anticoagulant rodenticide poisoning
Atrial fibrillation
Bacterial pneumonia
Blastomycosis
Blood loss anemia
Campylobacteriosis
Capillaria aerophilia infection
Cervical spondylomyelopathy (cervical
    vertebral instability, wobbler)
Cholangiohepatitis
Chronic bronchitis
Clostridial enteritis
Coccidioidomycosis
Congestive heart failure
Coronavirus enteritis
Cranial trauma
Crenosoma vulpis infection
Cryptococcosis
Cystic calculi
Cystitis
Degenerative myelopathy
Diabetes insipidus, central
Diabetes insipidus, nephrogenic
    (congenital)
Diabetes mellitus
Diabetic ketoacidosis
Dilated cardiomyopathy
Dirofilariasis
Disseminated intravascular coagulation
Distemper virus infection

Ehrlichia canis infection
Endocarditis—bacterial
Enteritis—bacterial
Epilepsy (idiopathic)
Exocrine pancreatic insufficiency
Feline immunodeficiency virus infection
Feline infectious peritonitis virus
    infection
Feline leukemia virus infection
Fibrocartilaginous embolism
Gastric antral mucosal hypertrophy
Gastric dilatation—volvulus
Gastric foreign body
Gastrointestinal parasitism
Gastrointestinal ulceration
Granulomatous meningoencephalitis
Hemangiosarcoma—atrial
Hemangiosarcoma—splenic
Hematoma—splenic
Hepatic cirrhosis
Hepatic disease
Hepatic encephalopathy
Hepatic lipidosis (idiopathic)
Hepatic neoplasia
Hepatitis (acute)
Hepatitis (chronic idiopathic)
Histoplasmosis
Hydrocephalus
Hyperadrenocorticism (adrenal adenoma
    or adenocarcinoma)
Hyperadrenocorticism, pituitary-
    dependent
Hypercalcemia
Hyperkalemia
Hyperlipidemia

PART

F

Hyperthyroidism
Hypertrophic cardiomyopathy
Hyperviscosity
Hypoadrenocorticism
Hypocalcemia
Hypoglycemia
Hypokalemia
Hypothyroidism
Hypoxia
Immune-mediated hemolytic anemia
Immune-mediated thrombocytopenia
Infectious tracheobronchitis
Inflammatory bowel disease
Intervertebral disk disease—cervical
Intervertebral disk disease—
    thoracolumbar
Intestinal obstruction (complete)
Intestinal obstruction (partial)
Intracranial disease
Lead toxicity
Lumbosacral vertebral canal stenosis
Lymphangiectasia
Lymphosarcoma—gastrointestinal
Lymphosarcoma—mediastinal
Lymphosarcoma—multicentric
Meningitis—bacterial
Meningitis—steroid-responsive (aseptic)
Myasthenia gravis
Narcolepsy
Neoplasia—bladder
Neoplasia—brain
Neoplasia—cardiac

Neoplasia—gastric
Neoplasia—intestinal
Neoplasia—nasal
Neoplasia—pulmonary
Oslerus (Filaroides) osleri infection
Pancreatitis (acute)
Parvoviral enteritis
Pericarditis
Peripheral neuropathy
Peritonitis
Pneumonia
Polycythemia vera
Polymyositis
Portosystemic shunt—congenital
Psychogenic polydipsia
Pulmonary edema
Pulmonary thromboembolism
Pyelonephritis
Pyloric stenosis
Pyometra
Renal failure, acute
Renal failure, chronic
Renal glucosuria (primary)
Rocky Mountain spotted fever
Salmonellosis
Small intestinal bacterial overgrowth
Tick paralysis
Toxoplasmosis
Urinary incontinence
Urolithiasis
Ventricular tachyarrhythmia
von Willebrand's disease

Section V

Part G
Treatment

PART G **Directions:** Select the treatment(s) you desire and look up the corresponding number(s) in the *Answers for Part G (Response to Therapy)*. Case summaries and explanations follow the answer section and are located at the end of the text.

To avoid bias and to make the case management exercise as realistic as possible, please read only the selected numbered answer.

DIETARY

Feeding via gastrostomy tube

Case 1=82	Case 2=1	Case 3=163	Case 4=1	Case 5=1	Case 6=1
Case 7=1	Case 8=1	Case 9=1	Case 10=82	Case 11=1	Case 12=241

Low-fat, high-fiber diet

Case 1=2	Case 2=2	Case 3=2	Case 4=2	Case 5=2	Case 6=2
Case 7=2	Case 8=2	Case 9=2	Case 10=83	Case 11=2	Case 12=164

Low-residue, highly digestible diet

Case 1=3	Case 2=3	Case 3=3	Case 4=3	Case 5=3	Case 6=3
Case 7=3	Case 8=3	Case 9=84	Case 10=165	Case 11=3	Case 12=242

Reduced-protein diet

Case 1=4	Case 2=4	Case 3=4	Case 4=4	Case 5=4	Case 6=4
Case 7=4	Case 8=4	Case 9=4	Case 10=243	Case 11=85	Case 12=166

PART

G

MEDICATIONS

Intravenous/parenteral medications

Amphotericin B administration

Case 1=5	Case 2=5	Case 3=5	Case 4=86	Case 5=5	Case 6=293
Case 7=5	Case 8=5	Case 9=5	Case 10=244	Case 11=5	Case 12=167

Atropine administration

Case 1=6	Case 2=6	Case 3=6	Case 4=6	Case 5=6	Case 6=6
Case 7=6	Case 8=6	Case 9=6	Case 10=87	Case 11=6	Case 12=6

Bicarbonate administration

Case 1=7	Case 2=380	Case 3=7	Case 4=7	Case 5=7	Case 6=7
Case 7=7	Case 8=7	Case 9=7	Case 10=88	Case 11=7	Case 12=7

Calcium administration—parenteral

Case 1=8	Case 2=8	Case 3=8	Case 4=8	Case 5=8	Case 6=8
Case 7=8	Case 8=8	Case 9=8	Case 10=245	Case 11=8	Case 12=89

Calcium ethylenediaminetetraacetic acid (EDTA) administration

Case 1=9	Case 2=9	Case 3=9	Case 4=9	Case 5=9	Case 6=9
Case 7=9	Case 8=9	Case 9=9	Case 10=90	Case 11=9	Case 12=168

Dexamethasone sodium phosphate administration—intravenous, one time

Case 1=10	Case 2=343	Case 3=246	Case 4=91	Case 5=169	Case 6=294
Case 7=10	Case 8=10	Case 9=10	Case 10=322	Case 11=10	Case 12=10

Diazepam administration

Case 1=247	Case 2=92	Case 3=11	Case 4=11	Case 5=11	Case 6=11
Case 7=11	Case 8=11	Case 9=11	Case 10=344	Case 11=170	Case 12=295

Dobutamine infusion

Case 1=296	Case 2=171	Case 3=324	Case 4=12	Case 5=12	Case 6=12
Case 7=12	Case 8=12	Case 9=12	Case 10=248	Case 11=12	Case 12=93

Glucose administration—intravenous

Case 1=172	Case 2=13	Case 3=13	Case 4=13	Case 5=13	Case 6=13
Case 7=249	Case 8=94	Case 9=13	Case 10=297	Case 11=13	Case 12=13

Heparin administration

Case 1=14	Case 2=323	Case 3=95	Case 4=14	Case 5=14	Case 6=14
Case 7=14	Case 8=14	Case 9=14	Case 10=173	Case 11=14	Case 12=250

Insulin administration

Case 1=15	Case 2=15	Case 3=15	Case 4=15	Case 5=15	Case 6=15
Case 7=15	Case 8=15	Case 9=15	Case 10=96	Case 11=15	Case 12=174

Lidocaine administration—intravenous

Case 1=97	Case 2=16	Case 3=16	Case 4=16	Case 5=16	Case 6=16
Case 7=16	Case 8=16	Case 9=16	Case 10=175	Case 11=16	Case 12=251

Melarsomine dihydrochloride administration

Case 1=18	Case 2=18	Case 3=18	Case 4=177	Case 5=18	Case 6=18
Case 7=18	Case 8=18	Case 9=18	Case 10=253	Case 11=18	Case 12=99

Prostaglandin $F_{2\alpha}$ administration

Case 1=17	Case 2=17	Case 3=17	Case 4=17	Case 5=17	Case 6=17
Case 7=17	Case 8=17	Case 9=98	Case 10=252	Case 11=17	Case 12=176

Vitamin K administration

Case 1=19	Case 2=19	Case 3=19	Case 4=19	Case 5=19	Case 6=19
Case 7=19	Case 8=19	Case 9=19	Case 10=100	Case 11=19	Case 12=178

Oral medications

Angiotensin converting enzyme (ACE) inhibitor (e.g., enalapril) administration

Case 1=20	Case 2=179	Case 3=20	Case 4=20	Case 5=20	Case 6=20
Case 7=20	Case 8=20	Case 9=20	Case 10=254	Case 11=20	Case 12=101

Ampicillin administration

Case 1=21	Case 2=21	Case 3=21	Case 4=21	Case 5=21	Case 6=21
Case 7=102	Case 8=21	Case 9=21	Case 10=255	Case 11=21	Case 12=180

Cephalexin administration

Case 1=103	Case 2=22	Case 3=22	Case 4=22	Case 5=22	Case 6=22
Case 7=298	Case 8=22	Case 9=22	Case 10=181	Case 11=22	Case 12=256

Cimetidine administration

Case 1=23	Case 2=23	Case 3=23	Case 4=23	Case 5=23	Case 6=23
Case 7=23	Case 8=23	Case 9=23	Case 10=182	Case 11=23	Case 12=104

Clindamycin administration

Case 1=24	Case 2=24	Case 3=24	Case 4=24	Case 5=24	Case 6=24
Case 7=24	Case 8=24	Case 9=24	Case 10=105	Case 11=24	Case 12=183

Colchicine administration

Case 1=25	Case 2=25	Case 3=25	Case 4=25	Case 5=25	Case 6=25
Case 7=25	Case 8=25	Case 9=25	Case 10=184	Case 11=25	Case 12=106

Diethylstilbesterol administration

Case 1=26	Case 2=26	Case 3=26	Case 4=26	Case 5=26	Case 6=26
Case 7=26	Case 8=26	Case 9=26	Case 10=107	Case 11=26	Case 12=185

Digoxin administration

Case 1=108	Case 2=27	Case 3=27	Case 4=27	Case 5=27	Case 6=27
Case 7=27	Case 8=27	Case 9=27	Case 10=186	Case 11=27	Case 12=257

Diltiazem administration

Case 1=28	Case 2=28	Case 3=28	Case 4=28	Case 5=28	Case 6=28
Case 7=28	Case 8=28	Case 9=28	Case 10=109	Case 11=28	Case 12=187

Doxycycline administration

Case 1=29	Case 2=29	Case 3=29	Case 4=29	Case 5=29	Case 6=29
Case 7=29	Case 8=29	Case 9=29	Case 10=188	Case 11=29	Case 12=110

Erythromycin administration

Case 1=30	Case 2=30	Case 3=30	Case 4=30	Case 5=30	Case 6=30
Case 7=30	Case 8=30	Case 9=30	Case 10=111	Case 11=30	Case 12=189

Fenbendazole administration

Case 1=31	Case 2=31	Case 3=31	Case 4=31	Case 5=112	Case 6=31
Case 7=31	Case 8=31	Case 9=31	Case 10=190	Case 11=31	Case 12=260

Fluconazole administration

Case 1=21	Case 2=32	Case 3=32	Case 4=32	Case 5=32	Case 6=191
Case 7=32	Case 8=32	Case 9=32	Case 10=261	Case 11=32	Case 12=113

Fludrocortisone administration

Case 1=114	Case 2=33	Case 3=33	Case 4=33	Case 5=33	Case 6=33
Case 7=325	Case 8=33	Case 9=33	Case 10=192	Case 11=33	Case 12=262

Furosemide administration

Case 1=193	Case 2=34	Case 3=34	Case 4=34	Case 5=34	Case 6=34
Case 7=115	Case 8=345	Case 9=263	Case 10=299	Case 11=34	Case 12=326

Hydroxyurea administration

Case 1=35	Case 2=35	Case 3=35	Case 4=35	Case 5=35	Case 6=35
Case 7=35	Case 8=35	Case 9=35	Case 10=116	Case 11=35	Case 12=194

Hypoglycemic medication administration (oral)

Case 1=36	Case 2=36	Case 3=36	Case 4=36	Case 5=36	Case 6=36
Case 7=36	Case 8=36	Case 9=36	Case 10=195	Case 11=36	Case 12=117

Itraconazole administration

Case 1=37	Case 2=37	Case 3=37	Case 4=37	Case 5=37	Case 6=37
Case 7=37	Case 8=37	Case 9=37	Case 10=118	Case 11=37	Case 12=196

Ketoconazole administration

Case 1=38	Case 2=38	Case 3=38	Case 4=38	Case 5=38	Case 6=300
Case 7=119	Case 8=197	Case 9=38	Case 10=327	Case 11=38	Case 12=264

Lactulose administration—oral

Case 1=39	Case 2=39	Case 3=39	Case 4=198	Case 5=39	Case 6=39
Case 7=120	Case 8=120	Case 9=346	Case 10=328	Case 11=265	Case 12=301

Methimazole administration

Case 1=40	Case 2=40	Case 3=40	Case 4=40	Case 5=40	Case 6=40
Case 7=40	Case 8=40	Case 9=40	Case 10=121	Case 11=40	Case 12=199

Metronidazole administration

Case 1=41	Case 2=41	Case 3=41	Case 4=41	Case 5=41	Case 6=41
Case 7=41	Case 8=41	Case 9=122	Case 10=200	Case 11=41	Case 12=41

Mitotane (o'p-DDD) administration

Case 1=43	Case 2=43	Case 3=43	Case 4=124	Case 5=43	Case 6=43
Case 7=302	Case 8=43	Case 9=43	Case 10=267	Case 11=43	Case 12=202

Neomycin administration

Case 1=42	Case 2=42	Case 3=42	Case 4=42	Case 5=42	Case 6=42
Case 7=42	Case 8=42	Case 9=42	Case 10=201	Case 11=123	Case 12=266

Pancreatic enzyme supplementation

Case 1=44	Case 2=44	Case 3=44	Case 4=44	Case 5=44	Case 6=44
Case 7=44	Case 8=44	Case 9=44	Case 10=125	Case 11=44	Case 12=203

Phenobarbital administration

Case 1=204	Case 2=45	Case 3=45	Case 4=268	Case 5=45	Case 6=45
Case 7=45	Case 8=45	Case 9=45	Case 10=329	Case 11=126	Case 12=303

Phenylpropanolamine administration

Case 1=46	Case 2=46	Case 3=46	Case 4=46	Case 5=46	Case 6=46
Case 7=46	Case 8=46	Case 9=46	Case 10=205	Case 11=46	Case 12=127

Potassium supplementation—oral

Case 1=47	Case 2=47	Case 3=47	Case 4=47	Case 5=47	Case 6=47
Case 7=47	Case 8=47	Case 9=47	Case 10=128	Case 11=47	Case 12=206

Prednisone administration

Case 1=304	Case 2=48	Case 3=379	Case 4=330	Case 5=376	Case 6=129
Case 7=370	Case 8=361	Case 9=207	Case 10=269	Case 11=48	Case 12=347

Procainamide administration

Case 1=130	Case 2=49	Case 3=49	Case 4=49	Case 5=49	Case 6=49
Case 7=49	Case 8=49	Case 9=49	Case 10=208	Case 11=49	Case 12=270

Pyridostigmine administration

Case 1=50	Case 2=50	Case 3=50	Case 4=271	Case 5=50	Case 6=50
Case 7=50	Case 8=50	Case 9=50	Case 10=209	Case 11=50	Case 12=131

Ranitidine administration

Case 1=51	Case 2=51	Case 3=51	Case 4=51	Case 5=51	Case 6=51
Case 7=51	Case 8=51	Case 9=51	Case 10=132	Case 11=51	Case 12=210

Sucralfate administration

Case 1=52	Case 2=52	Case 3=52	Case 4=52	Case 5=52	Case 6=52
Case 7=52	Case 8=52	Case 9=52	Case 10=211	Case 11=52	Case 12=133

Tetracycline administration

Case 1=53	Case 2=53	Case 3=53	Case 4=53	Case 5=53	Case 6=53
Case 7=53	Case 8=53	Case 9=53	Case 10=134	Case 11=53	Case 12=212

Thiazide diuretic administration

Case 1=54	Case 2=331	Case 3=54	Case 4=54	Case 5=54	Case 6=54
Case 7=213	Case 8=135	Case 9=54	Case 10=305	Case 11=54	Case 12=272

Thyroxine administration

Case 1=55	Case 2=55	Case 3=55	Case 4=55	Case 5=55	Case 6=55
Case 7=55	Case 8=55	Case 9=55	Case 10=214	Case 11=55	Case 12=136

Vitamin K administration

Case 1=19	Case 2=19	Case 3=19	Case 4=19	Case 5=19	Case 6=19
Case 7=19	Case 8=19	Case 9=19	Case 10=100	Case 11=19	Case 12=178

Other Medications

Cancer chemotherapy

Case 1=56	Case 2=371	Case 3=56	Case 4=362	Case 5=273	Case 6=306
Case 7=215	Case 8=137	Case 9=56	Case 10=332	Case 11=56	Case 12=348

Lactulose enema

Case 1=57	Case 2=57	Case 3=57	Case 4=216	Case 5=57	Case 6=57
Case 7=57	Case 8=57	Case 9=57	Case 10=138	Case 11=307	Case 12=274

Vasopressin administration (drops in conjunctival sac)

Case 1=58	Case 2=58	Case 3=58	Case 4=58	Case 5=58	Case 6=58
Case 7=58	Case 8=58	Case 9=58	Case 10=217	Case 11=58	Case 12=139

Miscellaneous treatment

Blood transfusion (whole, fresh)

Case 1=59	Case 2=308	Case 3=140	Case 4=59	Case 5=59	Case 6=59
Case 7=59	Case 8=59	Case 9=59	Case 10=275	Case 11=59	Case 12=218

Dip for ticks

Case 1=60	Case 2=60	Case 3=60	Case 4=60	Case 5=60	Case 6=60
Case 7=60	Case 8=60	Case 9=60	Case 10=219	Case 11=60	Case 12=141

Fluid therapy—intravenous, replacement type

Case 1=61	Case 2=381	Case 3=61	Case 4=61	Case 5=61	Case 6=61
Case 7=61	Case 8=61	Case 9=61	Case 10=220	Case 11=61	Case 12=142

Fluid therapy—intravenous, saline

Case 1=62	Case 2=143	Case 3=62	Case 4=62	Case 5=62	Case 6=62
Case 7=62	Case 8=62	Case 9=62	Case 10=221	Case 11=62	Case 12=277

Mannitol administration

Case 1=63	Case 2=222	Case 3=63	Case 4=63	Case 5=63	Case 6=63
Case 7=63	Case 8=63	Case 9=63	Case 10=144	Case 11=63	Case 12=278

No treatment

Case 1=279	Case 2=359	Case 3=145	Case 4=357	Case 5=309	Case 6=377
Case 7=372	Case 8=64	Case 9=349	Case 10=333	Case 11=223	Case 12=363

Nursing care/physical therapy

Case 1=65	Case 2=65	Case 3=65	Case 4=65	Case 5=65	Case 6=65
Case 7=65	Case 8=65	Case 9=65	Case 10=146	Case 11=65	Case 12=224

Oxygen (supplemental)

Case 1=66	Case 2=225	Case 3=66	Case 4=147	Case 5=66	Case 6=66
Case 7=66	Case 8=66	Case 9=66	Case 10=66	Case 11=384	Case 12=387

Pericardiocentesis

Case 1=67	Case 2=67	Case 3=148	Case 4=67	Case 5=67	Case 6=67
Case 7=67	Case 8=67	Case 9=67	Case 10=226	Case 11=385	Case 12=67

Phlebotomy—therapeutic

Case 1=68	Case 2=310	Case 3=149	Case 4=68	Case 5=68	Case 6=68
Case 7=68	Case 8=68	Case 9=68	Case 10=227	Case 11=68	Case 12=280

Plasma transfusion (fresh)

Case 1=69	Case 2=281	Case 3=69	Case 4=69	Case 5=69	Case 6=69
Case 7=69	Case 8=69	Case 9=69	Case 10=228	Case 11=69	Case 12=150

Thoracocentesis

Case 1=382	Case 2=382	Case 3=382	Case 4=383	Case 5=382	Case 6=382
Case 7=382	Case 8=382	Case 9=382	Case 10=386	Case 11=382	Case 12=382

Water restriction (gradual)

Case 1=70	Case 2=151	Case 3=70	Case 4=70	Case 5=70	Case 6=70
Case 7=311	Case 8=334	Case 9=229	Case 10=350	Case 11=70	Case 12=282

Surgical treatments

Adrenalectomy—bilateral

Case 1=71	Case 2=152	Case 3=364	Case 4=335	Case 5=71	Case 6=71
Case 7=230	Case 8=71	Case 9=351	Case 10=71	Case 11=283	Case 12=312

Adrenalectomy—unilateral

Case 1=72	Case 2=231	Case 3=365	Case 4=284	Case 5=313	Case 6=358
Case 7=336	Case 8=72	Case 9=373	Case 10=153	Case 11=352	Case 12=72

Cervical vertebral stabilization

Case 1=73	Case 2=73	Case 3=73	Case 4=154	Case 5=374	Case 6=378
Case 7=232	Case 8=337	Case 9=366	Case 10=314	Case 11=285	Case 12=353

Closure (surgical) of portosystemic shunt

Case 1=233	Case 2=367	Case 3=155	Case 4=354	Case 5=74	Case 6=74
Case 7=74	Case 8=74	Case 9=74	Case 10=286	Case 11=338	Case 12=315

Dorsal laminectomy to decompress the spinal cord

Case 1=75	Case 2=75	Case 3=75	Case 4=156	Case 5=316	Case 6=234
Case 7=75	Case 8=75	Case 9=75	Case 10=339	Case 11=234	Case 12=287

Hypophysectomy

Case 1=76	Case 2=76	Case 3=317	Case 4=235	Case 5=76	Case 6=76
Case 7=157	Case 8=76	Case 9=76	Case 10=288	Case 11=76	Case 12=76

Mass resection (surgical)

Case 1=77	Case 2=289	Case 3=77	Case 4=318	Case 5=77	Case 6=77
Case 7=77	Case 8=236	Case 9=77	Case 10=158	Case 11=77	Case 12=77

Ovariohysterectomy

Case 1=78	Case 2=375	Case 3=237	Case 4=355	Case 5=159	Case 6=78
Case 7=368	Case 8=78	Case 9=78	Case 10=340	Case 11=290	Case 12=319

Splenectomy

Case 1=320	Case 2=291	Case 3=341	Case 4=238	Case 5=79	Case 6=79
Case 7=79	Case 8=79	Case 9=79	Case 10=356	Case 11=369	Case 12=160

Thoracotomy

Case 1=80	Case 2=80	Case 3=360	Case 4=292	Case 5=321	Case 6=239
Case 7=161	Case 8=161	Case 9=161	Case 10=342	Case 11=161	Case 12=161

Thyroidectomy

Case 1=162	Case 2=81	Case 3=81	Case 4=81	Case 5=81	Case 6=81
Case 7=81	Case 8=81	Case 9=81	Case 10=162	Case 11=81	Case 12=240

Answers for Part G
(Response to Therapy)

1. Feeding via gastrostomy tube: no response

2. Low-fat, high-fiber diet: no response

3. Low-residue, highly digestible diet: no response

4. Reduced-protein diet: no response

5. Amphotericin B administration: No response. The dog develops acute renal failure 1 week after therapy has begun.

6. Atropine administration: the animal becomes tachycardic.

7. Intravenous bicarbonate administration: no response

8. Parenteral calcium administration: no response

9. Calcium ethylenediaminetetraacetic acid (EDTA) administration: no response

10. Dexamethasone phosphate (intravenous, one injection): no response

11. Diazepam administration: no improvement. The animal becomes lethargic.

12. Dobutamine infusion: no response

13. Glucose administration (intravenous): The animal becomes hyperglycemic and glucosuric. There is no improvement in the animal's condition.

14. Heparin administration: no response

15. Insulin therapy: you begin insulin therapy and keep the animal in the clinic the first day so that you can periodically check the blood glucose. This is fortunate, because despite the low dose of insulin, the animal becomes very hypoglycemic and has a seizure. You intravenously administer 5% dextrose in water for 12 hours until most of the insulin effects have worn off, and you then must explain to the animal's owners that you have concluded that their pet is not diabetic.

16. Intravenous lidocaine: no response

17. Prostaglandin $F_{2\alpha}$ administration: No response. In addition, the animal develops transient vomiting, diarrhea, and abdominal pain in response to the drug.

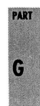

PART

G

18. Melarsomine dihydrochloride treatment: No response.

19. Vitamin K administration: no response

20. Angiotensin converting enzyme (ACE) inhibitor administration: no response

21. Ampicillin administration: no response

22. Cephalexin administration: no response

23. Cimetidine administration: no response

24. Clindamycin administration: no response

25. Colchicine administration: no response

26. Diethylstilbestrol administration: no response

27. Digoxin administration: No response. The animal begins to vomit and develops cardiac arrhythmias resulting from digoxin toxicity 5 days later.

28. Diltiazem administration: no response

29. Doxycycline administration: no response

30. Erythromycin administration: no response

31. Fenbendazole administration: no response

32. Fluconazole administration: no response

33. Fludrocortisone administration: no improvement

34. Furosemide administration: no response

35. Hydroxyurea administration: no response

36. Oral hypoglycemic medication administration: no response

37. Itraconazole treatment: no response

38. Ketoconazole administration: no response

39. Lactulose administration (per os): No response. The dog develops very liquid diarrhea.

40. Methimazole administration: no response

41. Metronidazole administration: no response

42. Neomycin (oral) administration: no response

43. Mitotane (o'p-DDD) administration: The dog develops drug-induced hypoadrenocorticism and is presented in shock 10 days later.

44. Pancreatic enzyme supplementation: no response

45. Phenobarbital administration: The dog becomes more lethargic and depressed.

46. Phenylpropanolamine administration: no response

47. Oral potassium administration: no response

48. Prednisone administration: no response

49. Procainamide administration: no response

50. Pyridostigmine (a cholinesterase inhibitor) administration: No response. The dog vomits intermittently and develops diarrhea due to drug administration. The owners take the dog to another clinic.

51. Ranitidine administration: no response

52. Sucralfate treatment: no response

53. Tetracycline administration: no response

54. Thiazide diuretic administration: no response

55. Thyroxine administration: no response

56. Cancer chemotherapy: No response. The dog develops severe neutropenia, vomiting, and diarrhea from the drug therapy.

57. Lactulose enema: No response. The dog bites your technician and she is out sick for a week.

58. Vasopressin administration: no response

59. Fresh whole blood transfusion: no response

60. Dip for ticks: no response

61. Intravenous fluid (replacement type) administration: no response

62. Intravenous saline administration: no response

63. Intravenous mannitol administration: no response

64. No treatment: The dog's signs progress and the dog is presented to an emergency clinic 2 weeks later because he is vomiting and unable to urinate. The owners file a complaint with the local veterinary medical association.

65. Nursing care/physical therapy: no response

66. Supplemental oxygen: no response

67. Pericardiocentesis: You obtain fresh blood and induce a paroxysm of ventricular tachycardia because there is no pericardial effusion and you have punctured the heart.

68. Therapeutic phlebotomy: no response

69. Fresh plasma administration: no response

70. Water restriction (gradual): The animal slowly becomes dehydrated and lethargic. The owners discontinue water restriction and take the animal to another veterinarian.

71. Adrenalectomy (bilateral): The dog experiences cardiac arrest during induction of general anesthesia. Cardiopulmonary resuscitation is unsuccessful.

72. Adrenalectomy (unilateral): The dog experiences cardiac arrest while under anesthesia. Cardiopulmonary resuscitation is unsuccessful. The owners are considering legal action.

73. Cervical vertebral stabilization: The dog experiences cardiac arrest while under anesthesia. Cardiopulmonary resuscitation is unsuccessful. The owners are considering legal action.

74. Surgical closure of portosystemic shunt: A shunt could not be identified.

75. Dorsal laminectomy: The dog experiences cardiac arrest while under anesthesia. Cardiopulmonary resuscitation is unsuccessful. The owners file a complaint with the state licensing board.

76. Hypophysectomy: The dog experiences cardiac arrest while under anesthesia. Cardiopulmonary resuscitation is unsuccessful. The owners are considering legal action.

77. Surgical resection of neoplastic mass: No such mass could be identified in this patient.

78. Ovariohysterectomy: Shortly after you begin exploring the abdomen, you notice that the dog is male and has been neutered. The owners plan to sue.

79. Splenectomy: The spleen is grossly and histologically normal. There is no improvement in the clinical signs. The owners are considering legal action.

80. Thoracotomy: The dog develops cardiac arrest during induction of general anesthesia for the thoracotomy. Cardiopulmonary resuscitation is unsuccessful.

81. Thyroidectomy: The animal's owners get a second opinion and find that there is no indication for a thyroidectomy in their pet. They file a complaint against you with the local veterinary medical association.

82. Feeding via gastrostomy tube: The dog goes into cardiac arrest during anesthetic induction for tube placement. Cardiopulmonary resuscitation is unsuccessful.

83. Low-fat, high-fiber diet: The dog will not eat. The dog goes into cardiac arrest 2 hours later and cannot be resuscitated.

84. Low-residue, highly digestible diet: The diarrhea episodes decrease slightly in severity and frequency, but fail to resolve completely.

85. Reduced-protein diet: The seizures decrease in severity and frequency but still occur.

86. Amphotericin B administration: No response. The cat develops acute renal failure 1 week after therapy has begun.

87. Atropine administration: No response. The dog goes into cardiac arrest 1 hour later and cannot be resuscitated.

88. Intravenous bicarbonate administration: The heart rate increases to 68 beats/min.

89. Parenteral calcium administration: No response. The lethargy and vomiting become worse.

90. Calcium ethylenediaminetetraacetic acid (EDTA) administration: No response. The dog goes into cardiac arrest 2 hours later and cannot be resuscitated.

91. Dexamethasone phosphate (intravenous, one injection): A transient (4 days) improvement in the dyspnea and demeanor occurs.

92. Diazepam administration: no improvement. The dog becomes more depressed.

93. Dobutamine infusion: No response. The lethargy and vomiting become worse.

94. Glucose administration (intravenous): The dog becomes hyperglycemic and glucosuric. There is no improvement in the hematuria or frequent urination.

95. Heparin administration: The epistaxis worsens.

96. Insulin therapy: If administered without concurrent intravenous glucose, the dog becomes extremely hypoglycemic, has several seizures, goes into cardiac arrest, and cannot be resuscitated. If administered with intravenous glucose, the heart rate increases to 68 beats/min and the dog regains some strength.

97. Intravenous lidocaine: Frequency and number of ventricular premature contractions decrease.

98. Prostaglandin $F_{2\alpha}$ administration: No response. In addition to the diarrhea, vomiting and abdominal pain are also seen in response to the drug.

99. Thiacetarsamide treatment: No response. The dog becomes icteric as a result of the medication and the lethargy and vomiting become worse.

100. Vitamin K administration: No response. The dog goes into cardiac arrest 2 hours later and cannot be resuscitated.

101. Angiotensin converting enzyme (ACE) inhibitor administration: No response. The lethargy and vomiting become worse.

102. Ampicillin administration: The polyuria decreases slightly but does not resolve.

103. Cephalexin administration: No response. The dog vomits intermittently due to drug administration and continues to have episodes of weakness.

104. Cimetidine administration: No response. The lethargy and vomiting become worse.

105. Clindamycin administration: No response. The dog goes into cardiac arrest 2 hours later and cannot be resuscitated.

106. Colchicine administration: No response. The lethargy and vomiting become worse.

107. Diethylstilbestrol administration: No response. The dog goes into cardiac arrest 2 hours later and cannot be resuscitated.

108. Digoxin administration: There is no observable response over the following month. The dog continues to have episodes of weakness.

109. Diltiazem administration: No response. The dog goes into cardiac arrest later that day and cannot be resuscitated.

110. Doxycycline administration: No response. The vomiting and lethargy become worse.

111. Erythromycin administration: No response. The dog goes into cardiac arrest 2 hours later and cannot be resuscitated.

112. Fenbendazole administration: Marked improvement after 5 days of therapy. The cough disappears within 1 week. The owners are thrilled and recommend you to all of their pet-owning friends.

113. Fluconazole administration: No response. The lethargy and vomiting become worse.

114. Fludrocortisone administration: no improvement. The owners are upset because the dog has become polyuric and polydipsic.

115. Furosemide administration: The problem becomes worse and the clients are irate.

116. Hydroxyurea administration: No response. The dog goes into cardiac arrest 2 hours later and cannot be resuscitated.

117. Oral hypoglycemic medication administration: No response. The lethargy and vomiting become worse.

118. Itraconazole treatment: No response. The dog goes into cardiac arrest 2 hours later and cannot be resuscitated.

119. Ketoconazole administration: After only a few days of treatment the polyuria resolves. The dog's owners are thrilled and they recommend you to all their pet-owning friends.

120. Lactulose administration (per os): No response. The owners are angry because the dog now has very liquid diarrhea in addition to the increased urination.

121. Methimazole administration: No response. The dog goes into cardiac arrest 2 hours later and cannot be resuscitated.

122. Metronidazole administration: The diarrhea resolves more quickly than with previous episodes. No new episodes occur for three and one-half weeks, but then mild diarrhea recurs.

123. Neomycin (oral) administration: The dog seems more alert and active.

124. Mitotane (o′p-DDD) administration: No response. The cat begins vomiting as a side effect of the drug. The owners take the cat to another clinic.

125. Pancreatic enzyme supplementation: The dog is anorexic and will not eat the enzymes with food. The dog goes into cardiac arrest 2 hours later and cannot be resuscitated.

126. Phenobarbital administration: The dog becomes profoundly depressed and almost comatose.

127. Phenylpropanolamine administration: No response. The vomiting and lethargy become worse.

128. Oral potassium administration: The dog goes into cardiac arrest 30 minutes later and cannot be resuscitated.

129. Prednisone administration: The dog is brighter and more alert the next day; however, 3 days later the dog becomes more depressed and progresses into a coma.

130. Procainamide administration: Decreases but does not eliminate the ventricular tachyarrhythmia. The episodes of weakness become less frequent. Six months later the dog develops signs of congestive heart failure resulting from the underlying dilated cardiomyopathy. The owners are pleased with your efforts and recommend you to their pet-owning friends.

131. Pyridostigmine (a cholinesterase inhibitor) administration: No response. The vomiting and lethargy become worse.

132. Ranitidine administration: No response. The dog goes into cardiac arrest 2 hours later and cannot be resuscitated.

133. Sucralfate administration: The dog vomits the sucralfate shortly after administration. The lethargy and vomiting become worse.

134. Tetracycline administration: No response. The dog goes into cardiac arrest 2 hours later and cannot be resuscitated.

135. Thiazide diuretic administration: Now the dog is also urinating large volumes. The owners are not pleased.

136. Thyroxine administration: No response. The lethargy and vomiting become worse.

137. Cancer chemotherapy: Partial remission occurs and the dog's clinical signs decrease in severity for several weeks. The remission is only temporary, however, and the tumor begins to grow again, ultimately obstructing the urethra. The dog is euthanized. Despite the outcome, the dog's owners are very pleased about the added time they gained with their pet as a result of your treatment, and make a donation in your name to your alma mater.

138. Lactulose enema: No response. The dog goes into cardiac arrest 1 hour later and cannot be resuscitated.

139. Vasopressin administration: No response. The lethargy and vomiting become worse.

140. Fresh whole blood transfusion: The dog becomes polycythemic, and the epistaxis ceases for 24 hours but then begins again.

141. Dip for ticks: No response. The lethargy and vomiting become worse.

142. Intravenous fluid (replacement type) administration: The mucous membranes become less tacky, but the lethargy and vomiting persist and slowly become worse.

143. Intravenous saline: Mucous membrane pallor, capillary refill time, mental alertness, and strength improve over the next several hours. The dog is stable and doing much better 24 hours later.

144. Intravenous mannitol administration: The dog becomes more hypovolemic and shows worsening signs of shock. Cardiac arrest occurs and resuscitation is unsuccessful.

145. No treatment: The dog continues to bleed from the nose. The owners take the dog to another clinic.

146. Nursing care/physical therapy: No response. The dog goes into cardiac arrest 1 hour later and cannot be resuscitated.

147. Supplemental oxygen: The cat is more comfortable and less anxious.

148. Pericardiocentesis: You obtain fresh blood and induce a paroxysm of ventricular tachycardia because there is no pericardial effusion and you have punctured the heart. Hemorrhage continues into the pericardial sac and the dog develops acute cardiac tamponade and dies.

149. Therapeutic phlebotomy: excessive hemorrhage occurs at the venipuncture site and the dog's condition is not improved.

150. Fresh plasma administration: No response. The lethargy and vomiting become worse.

151. Water restriction (gradual): The signs of shock continue and the dog dies.

152. Adrenalectomy (bilateral): After you have removed the adrenal glands, you notice a splenic mass.

153. Adrenalectomy (unilateral): The dog goes into cardiac arrest during anesthetic induction and cannot be resuscitated.

154. Cervical vertebral stabilization: The cat experiences cardiac arrest while under anesthesia. Cardiopulmonary resuscitation is unsuccessful. The owners are considering legal action.

155. Surgical closure of portosystemic shunt: A shunt could not be identified. Excessive bleeding occurs throughout and after the procedure. Multiple blood transfusions are required.

156. Dorsal laminectomy: The cat experiences cardiac arrest while under anesthesia. Cardiopulmonary resuscitation is unsuccessful. The owners file a complaint with the state licensing board.

157. Hypophysectomy: Although a possible treatment, you are not equipped or trained to do a hypophysectomy and neither is anyone in your area. Please choose another treatment.

158. Surgical resection of neoplastic mass: A mass is not identified in the patient. The dog goes into cardiac arrest while under anesthesia and cannot be resuscitated.

159. Ovariohysterectomy: The uterus is grossly and histologically normal. The cough continues.

160. Splenectomy: The spleen is grossly normal, but a large fluid-filled uterus is found when the abdomen is explored.

161. Thoracotomy: The owners take the dog to another clinic and find that there is no need for a thoracotomy. They file a complaint with the state licensing board.

162. Thyroidectomy: The dog goes into cardiac arrest during anesthetic induction and cannot be resuscitated.

163. Feeding via gastrostomy tube: The dog bleeds excessively during and after placement of the tube, and ultimately requires a blood transfusion.

164. Low-fat, high-fiber diet: The dog will not eat. The vomiting and lethargy become worse.

165. Low-residue, highly digestible diet: The dog will not eat. The dog goes into cardiac arrest later that evening and cannot be resuscitated.

166. Reduced protein diet: The dog will not eat. The lethargy and vomiting become worse.

167. Amphotericin B administration: No response. The lethargy and vomiting become worse.

168. Calcium ethylenediaminetetraacetic acid (EDTA) administration: No response. The vomiting and lethargy become worse.

169. Dexamethasone phosphate (intravenous, one injection): A marked but transient improvement occurs; within 10 days, however, the dog is back to its pretreatment state.

170. Diazepam administration: The dog becomes extremely depressed and lethargic.

171. Dobutamine infusion: A transient improvement in mucous membrane color and capillary refill time is observed.

172. Glucose administration (intravenous): The dog becomes hyperglycemic and glucosuric, and still has episodes of weakness after he is discharged. The owners take the dog to another clinic.

173. Heparin administration: No response. The dog goes into cardiac arrest 2 hours later and cannot be resuscitated.

174. Insulin therapy: The dog becomes hypoglycemic and has several seizures. The lethargy and vomiting become worse.

175. Intravenous lidocaine: No response. The dog goes into cardiac arrest 30 minutes later and cannot be resuscitated.

176. Prostaglandin $F_{2\alpha}$ administration: After administration of the first dose, you notice mucopurulent material dripping from the vulva. If prostaglandin $F_{2\alpha}$ injections are your only treatment, the dog develops sepsis by the following day and dies despite intensive care. If you used this in conjunction with antibiotic treatment and other supportive care, the dog slowly improves over the next several days. (Note: There is a risk of uterine rupture [and resultant septic peritonitis] when prostaglandin $F_{2\alpha}$ is used to treat a closed-cervix pyometra. It is also not recommended in a dog with systemic signs of illness due to the pyometra. Thus, it is not the optimal treatment for this patient [you were lucky that the cervix opened versus the uterus rupturing]. Ovariohysterectomy with concurrent antibiotic treatment and supportive care is the treatment of choice.)

177. Melarsomine dihydrochloride treatment: The cat's dyspnea worsens, and it dies 3 hours later.

178. Vitamin K administration: No response. The lethargy and vomiting become worse.

179. Angiotensin converting enzyme (ACE) inhibitor administration: The dog becomes more hypotensive and progresses further into shock.

180. Ampicillin administration: The dog's clinical deterioration slows, but the clinical signs persist.

181. Cephalexin administration: No response. The dog goes into cardiac arrest 2 hours later and cannot be resuscitated.

182. Cimetidine administration: No response. The dog goes into cardiac arrest 2 hours later and cannot be resuscitated.

183. Clindamycin administration: No response. The vomiting and lethargy become worse.

184. Colchicine administration: No response. The dog goes into cardiac arrest 2 hours later and cannot be resuscitated.

185. Diethylstilbestrol administration: No response. The vomiting and lethargy become worse.

186. Digoxin administration: No response. The dog goes into cardiac arrest 1 hour later and cannot be resuscitated.

187. Diltiazem administration: No response. The lethargy and vomiting become worse.

188. Doxycycline administration: No response. The dog goes into cardiac arrest 2 hours later and cannot be resuscitated.

189. Erythromycin administration: No response. The vomiting and lethargy become worse.

190. Fenbendazole administration: No response. The dog goes into cardiac arrest later that evening and cannot be resuscitated.

191. Fluconazole administration: The dog improves steadily over the next several days and becomes clinically normal in several weeks.

192. Fludrocortisone administration: The dog improves dramatically. Two days later she is back to her usual attitude and activity. The owners recommend you to all their pet-owning friends!

193. Furosemide administration: There is no observable benefit and the episodes of weakness continue. The owners are somewhat annoyed because the dog has begun urinating in the house.

194. Hydroxyurea administration: No response. The vomiting and lethargy become worse.

195. Oral hypoglycemic medication administration: No response. The dog goes into cardiac arrest 2 hours later and cannot be resuscitated.

196. Itraconazole treatment: No response. The lethargy and vomiting become worse.

197. Ketoconazole administration: After 4 days of treatment the dog stops eating and beings vomiting. Results of an adrenocorticotropic hormone (ACTH) stimulation test show that the dog is glucocorticoid-deficient. The dog responds well to discontinuation of the ketoconazole and supplementation with low-dose prednisone for several days. However, the original clinical signs are still present and the treatment costs are mounting.

198. Lactulose administration (per os): No response. The cat develops very liquid diarrhea.

199. Methimazole administration: No response. The vomiting and lethargy become worse.

200. Metronidazole administration: No response. The dog goes into cardiac arrest 2 hours later and cannot be resuscitated.

201. Neomycin (oral) administration: No response. The dog goes into cardiac arrest 2 hours later and cannot be resuscitated.

202. Mitotane (o'p-DDD) administration: No response. The dog is returned to your clinic 16 hours later with overwhelming sepsis and dies despite intensive care.

203. Pancreatic enzyme supplementation: The dog vomits the food and enzyme mixture. The lethargy and vomiting become worse.

204. Phenobarbital administration: No response. The episodes of weakness continue. The owners are concerned over the drug-induced lethargy and polyphagia.

205. Phenylpropanolamine administration: No response. The dog goes into cardiac arrest 2 hours later and cannot be resuscitated.

206. Oral potassium administration: The dog vomits the oral potassium.

207. Prednisone administration: There is marked improvement. The diarrhea episode resolves and the dog passes the 6-week mark without another episode. The owners make a donation in your name to your alma mater.

208. Procainamide administration: The bradycardia and weakness become worse. The dog goes into cardiac arrest 1 hour later and cannot be resuscitated.

209. Pyridostigmine (a cholinesterase inhibitor) administration: The bradycardia and weakness become worse. The dog goes into cardiac arrest and cardiopulmonary resuscitation is unsuccessful.

210. Ranitidine administration: No response. The vomiting and lethargy become worse.

211. Sucralfate treatment: No response. The dog goes into cardiac arrest 2 hours later and cannot be resuscitated.

212. Tetracycline administration: No response. The lethargy and vomiting become worse.

213. Thiazide diuretic administration: The polyuria is worse. The dog's owners are becoming frustrated with getting out of bed several times each night to let the dog go outside.

214. Thyroxine administration: No response. The dog goes into cardiac arrest 2 hours later and cannot be resuscitated.

215. Cancer chemotherapy: The owners go to another veterinarian for a second opinion and find that their dog does not have cancer. They file a complaint with the local veterinary medical association.

216. Lactulose enema: No response. The cat bites your technician and she is out sick for a week.

217. Vasopressin administration: No response. The dog goes into cardiac arrest 2 hours later and cannot be resuscitated.

218. Fresh whole blood transfusion: No response. The vomiting and lethargy become worse.

219. Dip for ticks: The dog struggles slightly as it is being placed in the tub. The bradycardia becomes worse and the dog goes into cardiac arrest. Cardiopulmonary resuscitation is unsuccessful.

220. Intravenous fluid (replacement type) administration: The femoral pulses become stronger and the dog is a bit stronger, but the other signs persist and the dog is still unable or unwilling to stand.

221. Intravenous saline administration: The heart rate increases to 72 beats/min and the weakness is not as severe.

222. Intravenous mannitol: The signs of hypovolemia and shock worsen as the animal loses fluid because of a mannitol-induced osmotic diuresis.

223. No treatment: The seizures become more frequent. Two months later additional neurologic deficits develop and the dog lapses into a coma.

224. Nursing care/physical therapy: No response. The lethargy and vomiting become worse.

225. Supplemental oxygen: The dog seems to be slightly more comfortable.

226. Pericardiocentesis: You obtain fresh blood because there is no pericardial effusion and you have punctured the heart. The dog goes into cardiac arrest and cannot be resuscitated.

227. Therapeutic phlebotomy: The dog's shock and hypovolemia worsen. Cardiac arrest occurs and resuscitation is unsuccessful.

228. Fresh plasma administration: No response. The dog goes into cardiac arrest 2 hours later and cannot be resuscitated.

229. Water restriction (gradual): The dog becomes dehydrated because of the continuing diarrhea in conjunction with water restriction and is returned to your clinic. Intravenous rehydration is needed. The owners are not pleased.

230. Adrenalectomy (bilateral): The surgery goes well. Initial postoperative treatment of the dog's hypoadrenocorticism is challenging but successful. The dog returns to her normal routine and does well as long as she is continued on fludrocortisone and prednisone treatment. (Although bilateral adrenalectomy is an acceptable treatment for pituitary dependent hyperadrenocorticism, medical treatment of the disorder is effective, and is also less invasive and less costly.)

231. Adrenalectomy (unilateral): After you have removed the adrenal gland, you notice a splenic mass.

232. Cervical vertebral stabilization: The dog develops postoperative vertebral osteomyelitis and the polyuria continues. The owners are considering legal action.

233. Surgical closure of portosystemic shunt: The dog experiences cardiac arrest while under anesthesia. Cardiopulmonary resuscitation is unsuccessful. The owners are considering legal action.

234. Dorsal laminectomy: There are no abnormal findings during surgery. The dog develops severe postoperative neurologic deficits, lapses into a coma, and dies 1 day later.

235. Hypophysectomy: The cat experiences cardiac arrest while under anesthesia. Cardiopulmonary resuscitation is unsuccessful. The owners are considering legal action.

236. Surgical resection of neoplastic mass: A friable mass in the trigone area of the bladder cannot be completely resected without damaging the ureteral openings to the bladder, but you obtain a biopsy. Histopathology shows the mass to be transitional cell carcinoma.

237. Ovariohysterectomy: You cannot find the uterus because the dog was spayed years ago. Excessive hemorrhage occurs during surgery and multiple blood transfusions are required.

238. Splenectomy: The cat experiences cardiac arrest while under anesthesia. Cardiopulmonary resuscitation is unsuccessful. The owners are considering legal action.

239. Thoracotomy: No abnormalities are identified. The dog never fully recovers from general anesthesia, lapses into a coma, and dies.

240. Thyroidectomy: The dog's owners take the dog to another clinic for a second opinion and find there is no indication for a thyroidectomy in their dog. The other clinic makes the correct diagnosis and successfully treats the dog. The owners file a complaint against you with the local veterinary medical association.

241. Feeding via gastrostomy tube: The dog vomits any food it is fed. The lethargy and vomiting continue.

242. Low-residue, highly digestible diet: The dog will not eat. The lethargy and vomiting become worse.

243. Reduced protein diet: The dog will not eat. The dog goes into cardiac arrest 2 hours later and cannot be resuscitated.

244. Amphotericin B administration: No response. The dog goes into cardiac arrest later that evening and cannot be resuscitated.

245. Parenteral calcium administration: The heart rate increases to 64 beats/min.

246. Dexamethasone phosphate (intravenous, one injection): no response; epistaxis and thrombocytopenia continue

247. Diazepam administration: No response. The owners complain that the dog is listless while on the medication.

248. Dobutamine infusion: No response. The dog goes into cardiac arrest 2 hours later and cannot be resuscitated.

249. Glucose administration (intravenous): The dog becomes hyperglycemic and glucosuric. The increase in urination is worse.

250. Heparin administration: No response. The lethargy and vomiting become worse.

251. Intravenous lidocaine: No response. The lethargy and vomiting become worse.

252. Prostaglandin $F_{2\alpha}$ administration: No response. The dog goes into cardiac arrest 1 hour later and cannot be resuscitated.

253. Melarsomine dihydrochloride treatment: No response. The dog goes into cardiac arrest 2 hours later and cannot be resuscitated.

254. Angiotensin converting enzyme (ACE) inhibitor administration: No response. The dog goes into cardiac arrest 2 hours later and cannot be resuscitated.

255. Ampicillin administration: No response. The dog goes into cardiac arrest 2 hours later and cannot be resuscitated.

256. Cephalexin administration: The dog's fever decreases, but the dog remains very ill.

257. Digoxin administration: No response. The vomiting and lethargy become worse.

258. Diltiazem administration: no response.

259. Doxycycline administration: no response.

260. Fenbendazole administration: The dog vomits the medication.

261. Fluconazole administration: No response. The dog goes into cardiac arrest later that evening and cannot be resuscitated.

262. Fludrocortisone administration: No improvement. The dog develops overwhelming sepsis and dies despite intensive treatment.

263. Furosemide administration: The owners are upset because now the dog is urinating frequently in addition to having diarrhea.

264. Ketoconazole administration: No response. The lethargy and vomiting become worse.

265. Lactulose administration (per os): The seizures decrease in frequency and severity. The owners also report that the dog is more alert and playful.

266. Neomycin (oral) administration: No response. The lethargy and vomiting become worse.

267. Mitotane (o'p-DDD) administration: The dog goes into cardiac arrest later that evening and cannot be resuscitated.

268. Phenobarbital administration: The cat becomes more lethargic and depressed.

269. Prednisone administration: The dog improves slightly. She is brighter, begins to eat again, and is strong enough to lie sternally.

270. Procainamide administration: No improvement. The vomiting and lethargy become worse.

271. Pyridostigmine (a cholinesterase inhibitor) administration: No response. The cat begins to vomit intermittently and develops diarrhea due to drug administration. The owners take the cat to another clinic.

272. Thiazide diuretic administration: No response. The lethargy and vomiting become worse.

273. Cancer chemotherapy: The frequency of the cough is reduced; however, the dog develops severe neutropenia, vomiting, and diarrhea from the drug therapy.

274. Lactulose enema: No response. The lethargy and vomiting become worse.

275. Fresh whole blood transfusion: No response. The dog goes into cardiac arrest 2 hours later and cannot be resuscitated.

276. Intravenous fluid (replacement type) administration: Mucous membrane pallor, capillary refill time, mental alertness, and strength improve over the next several hours. The dog is stable and doing much better 24 hours later.

277. Intravenous saline administration: The mucous membranes become less tacky, but the lethargy and vomiting persist and slowly become worse.

278. Intravenous mannitol administration: The dog becomes more dehydrated and the lethargy and vomiting become worse.

279. No treatment: The dog continues to have episodes of weakness. Two months later, the owners call to tell you the dog "dropped dead" in the backyard yesterday, and that they are planning to sue.

280. Therapeutic phlebotomy: The mucous membranes become tackier. The lethargy and vomiting become worse.

281. Fresh plasma administration: The dog is slow to respond, but is stronger and brighter 24 hours later.

282. Water restriction (gradual): The dog becomes dehydrated because of continued vomiting in conjunction with water restriction. The clinical signs become worse over the following 12 hours and the dog is returned to your clinic with overwhelming sepsis. Cardiac arrest occurs despite intensive care.

283. Adrenalectomy (bilateral): The surgery goes well, but the dog has a prolonged anesthetic recovery. The seizures continue, and the owners now have to treat the iatrogenic hypoadrenocorticism. The dog's owners are not pleased and file a complaint with the local veterinary medical association.

284. Adrenalectomy (unilateral): The cat's dyspnea continues postoperatively and it dies within 24 hours.

285. Cervical vertebral stabilization: The dog has a prolonged anesthetic recovery. She develops postoperative vertebral osteomyelitis and the seizures continue. The owners are considering legal action.

286. Surgical closure of portosystemic shunt: The dog goes into cardiac arrest during anesthetic induction and cannot be resuscitated.

287. Dorsal laminectomy: There are no abnormal findings during surgery. The clinical signs become worse and the dog goes into cardiac arrest the following day; cardiopulmonary resuscitation is unsuccessful.

288. Hypophysectomy: The dog goes into cardiac arrest during anesthetic induction and cannot be resuscitated.

289. Surgical resection of neoplastic mass: The dog recovers well from the surgery and lives another 5 months before the tumor recurs in the liver. The dog is euthanized at that time. The owners are very pleased with your efforts.

290. Ovariohysterectomy: The surgery goes well, but the dog has a prolonged anesthetic recovery. The seizures continue.

291. Splenectomy: The dog recovers well from the surgery and lives another 5 months before the tumor recurs in the liver. The dog is euthanized at that time. The owners are very pleased with your efforts.

292. Thoracotomy: A cranial mediastinal mass is identified during surgery. Biopsy results reveal lymphosarcoma. The cat develops pyothorax postoperatively due to a nosocomial infection with *Pseudomonas aeruginosa,* which proves fatal.

293. Amphotericin B administration: The dog's signs improve after two treatments. However, acute renal failure develops after three treatments and drug administration is stopped.

294. Dexamethasone phosphate (intravenous, one injection): The dog's signs improve for 2 days, then the dogs lapses into a coma and dies.

295. Diazepam administration: no improvement. The lethargy and vomiting become worse.

296. Dobutamine infusion: exacerbates the ventricular tachyarrhythmia resulting in frequent syncopal episodes

297. Glucose administration (intravenous): The dog's heart rate increases to 68 beats/min and the dog is a little stronger.

298. Cephalexin administration: The polyuria decreases but is still present.

299. Furosemide administration: No response. The bradycardia and weakness become worse and the dog goes into cardiac arrest 1 hour later. Cardiopulmonary resuscitation is unsuccessful.

300. Ketoconazole administration: The dog improves slowly over the next several weeks, but then relapses.

301. Lactulose administration (per os): The dog vomits the medication. The lethargy and vomiting become worse.

302. Mitotane (o'p-DDD) administration: Happy clients! After only a few days of treatment the polyuria decreases, and urination is back to normal within 10 days. They recommend you to all their pet-owning friends.

303. Phenobarbital administration: No response. The lethargy and vomiting become worse.

304. Prednisone administration: No response. The owners are upset with the drug-induced polyuria and polydipsia. The episodes of weakness continue.

305. Thiazide diuretic administration: No response. The dog goes into cardiac arrest 2 hours later and cannot be resuscitated.

306. Cancer chemotherapy: The dog improves for a few days, then lapses into a coma and dies.

307. Lactulose enema: The dog seems more alert and more active.

308. Fresh whole blood transfusion: The dog responds to therapy and is much brighter and stronger 24 hours later.

309. No treatment: The cough continues.

310. Therapeutic phlebotomy: The dog's shock worsens and it dies. The owners are considering legal action.

311. Water restriction (gradual): The polyuria continues despite gradual water restriction. The dog drinks all the water she is given and begs for more, also attempting to drink from peoples' glasses and cups. She then becomes lethargic and is presented to your clinic, where she is found to be at least 7% dehydrated. You rehydrate her over the next 6–12 hours, and she returns to her normal attitude. The dog's owners are quite upset and remark, "Obviously water restriction is **not** what's needed!"

312. Adrenalectomy (bilateral): You find a large, fluid-filled uterus when you open the abdomen for the adrenalectomy.

313. Adrenalectomy (unilateral): The dog's cough is not improved following surgery and the owners question the need for surgery. They are considering legal action.

314. Cervical vertebral stabilization: The dog goes into cardiac arrest during anesthetic induction and cannot be resuscitated.

315. Surgical closure of portosystemic shunt: No shunt is identified, but a large, fluid-filled uterus is observed when the abdomen is explored.

316. Dorsal laminectomy: There are no abnormal findings during surgery. The dog develops postoperative neurologic deficits, and continues to cough.

317. Hypophysectomy: Excessive bleeding occurs during surgery, and the dog experiences cardiac arrest while under anesthesia. Cardiopulmonary resuscitation is unsuccessful. The owners are considering legal action.

318. Surgical resection of neoplastic mass: The cat experiences cardiac arrest shortly after anesthesia induction. Cardiopulmonary resuscitation is unsuccessful.

319. Ovariohysterectomy: You find a large, hyperemic, fluid-filled uterus. The ovariohysterectomy is successful. The dog improves dramatically, especially if also treated with intravenous fluids and antibiotics.

320. Splenectomy: The dog experiences cardiac arrest while under anesthesia. Cardiopulmonary resuscitation is unsuccessful. The owners are considering legal action.

321. Thoracotomy: No abnormalities are identified. The dog continues to cough until it chews off its chest tube and dies of acute pneumothorax 1 day after surgery.

322. Dexamethasone phosphate (intravenous, one injection): The dog's heart rate increases to near normal, her strength improves, and she begins eating again; however, 24 hours later the signs begin to recur.

323. Heparin administration: The dog's condition deteriorates and he dies 6 hours later.

324. Dobutamine infusion: The epistaxis continues and the dog develops ventricular arrhythmias during the infusion.

325. Fludrocortisone administration: The polyuria becomes worse.

326. Furosemide administration: no improvement. The vomiting and lethargy get worse.

327. Ketoconazole administration: No response. The dog goes into cardiac arrest later that evening and cannot be resuscitated.

328. Lactulose administration (per os): no improvement. The dog goes into cardiac arrest later that evening and cannot be resuscitated.

329. Phenobarbital administration: The bradycardia becomes worse and the dog goes into cardiac arrest 2 hours later. Cardiopulmonary resuscitation is unsuccessful.

330. Prednisone administration: The cat begins to feel much better and the dyspnea is reduced. However, the cat is returned in 3 weeks with severe dyspnea.

331. Thiazide diuretic administration: exacerbates the hypovolemia present in this dog

332. Cancer chemotherapy: You plan to initiate chemotherapy the following morning, but the dog goes into cardiac arrest that evening and cannot be resuscitated.

333. No treatment: The dog goes into cardiac arrest 2 hours later and cannot be resuscitated.

334. Water restriction (gradual): The owners are unable to restrict the dog's water intake without drastically altering their and the dog's lifestyle. They also do not believe that excess intake is causing the problem because the dog only urinates a small amount each time. (The owners are correct!)

335. Adrenalectomy (bilateral): Cardiac arrest occurs while the cat is under general anesthesia. Cardiopulmonary resuscitation is unsuccessful.

336. Adrenalectomy (unilateral): The adrenalectomy goes well but the polyuria persists. The dog's owners are not pleased.

337. Cervical vertebral stabilization: The dog develops postoperative vertebral osteomyelitis and the pollakiuria continues. The owners are considering legal action.

338. Surgical closure of portosystemic shunt: The surgery is a success. The owners are thrilled because the dog is more alert, active, and playful than she had ever been. They recommend you to all their pet-owning friends!

339. Dorsal laminectomy: The dog goes into cardiac arrest during anesthetic induction and cannot be resuscitated.

340. Ovariohysterectomy: The dog goes into cardiac arrest during anesthetic induction and cannot be resuscitated. The owners plan to sue because the dog was spayed several months earlier.

341. Splenectomy: The dog bleeds excessively during surgery and becomes very anemic. Multiple blood transfusions are given over the next week. Eventually the dog recovers and the platelet count increases but not to normal. Although splenectomy can be used to treat immune-related thrombocytopenia, immunosuppressive drug therapy (i.e., prednisone) is preferred unless the animal becomes refractory to all treatments.

342. Thoracotomy: The dog goes into cardiac arrest during anesthetic induction and cannot be resuscitated.

343. Dexamethasone phosphate (intravenous, one injection): If given with no other therapy, there is no response; however, if administered in conjunction with intravenous fluids, it helps reverse the shock state.

344. Diazepam administration: no improvement. The dog goes into cardiac arrest 2 hours later and cannot be resuscitated.

345. Furosemide administration: The problem is worse. Now the dog urinates larger volumes in addition to urinating often.

346. Lactulose administration (per os): No response; in fact, the diarrhea seems worse.

347. Prednisone administration: The dog becomes more depressed and the vomiting is worse. She becomes septic and dies despite intensive care.

348. Cancer chemotherapy: No response. The dog develops overwhelming sepsis and dies despite intensive care.

349. No treatment: The diarrhea episodes continue and the diarrhea is now accompanied by vomiting. The owners take the dog to another clinic.

350. Water restriction (gradual): The dog goes into cardiac arrest 2 hours later and cannot be resuscitated.

351. Adrenalectomy (bilateral): The surgery goes well, but the diarrhea episodes continue and the dog now requires treatment for the iatrogenic hypoadrenocorticism. The dog's owners are not pleased and file a complaint with the local veterinary medical association.

352. Adrenalectomy (unilateral): The surgery goes well, but the dog has a prolonged anesthetic recovery. The seizures continue.

353. Cervical vertebral stabilization: No improvement. The clinical signs become worse and the following day the dog goes into cardiac arrest. Cardiopulmonary resuscitation is unsuccessful. The owners are considering legal action.

354. Surgical closure of portosystemic shunt: A shunt could not be identified. The cat experiences cardiac arrest during anesthesia. Cardiopulmonary resuscitation is unsuccessful. The owners plan to sue.

355. Ovariohysterectomy: The cat experiences cardiac arrest during anesthesia. Cardiopulmonary resuscitation is unsuccessful. The owners plan to sue.

356. Splenectomy: The dog goes into cardiac arrest during anesthetic induction and cannot be resuscitated.

357. No treatment: The cat dies at home 1 week later.

358. Adrenalectomy (unilateral): The dog's condition deteriorates postoperatively. It becomes comatose and dies 12 hours later.

359. No treatment: The dog dies 3 hours later. The owners are planning to sue.

360. Thoracotomy: The dog develops severe hemorrhage during surgery and dies despite fluid therapy and a blood transfusion.

361. Prednisone administration: The problem is worse. Now the dog urinates large amounts in addition to urinating often.

362. Cancer chemotherapy: The cat tolerates the therapy well and has a good quality of life for another 8 months until the lymphosarcoma recurs. The owners were pleased with your efforts.

363. No treatment: The dog's signs quickly become worse and the dog is presented to an emergency clinic the following day with overwhelming sepsis. They make the correct diagnosis (pyometra) and treat her appropriately. She recovers, but only with intensive care. The owners are planning to sue.

364. Adrenalectomy (bilateral): Excessive hemorrhage occurs during surgery and the dog dies despite aggressive intravenous fluid therapy and a blood transfusion.

365. Adrenalectomy (unilateral): Severe hemorrhage and cardiac arrest occur while the dog is under anesthesia. Cardiopulmonary resuscitation is unsuccessful. The owners are considering legal action.

366. Cervical vertebral stabilization: The dog develops postoperative vertebral osteomyelitis and the diarrhea continues. The owners are considering legal action.

367. Surgical closure of portosystemic shunt: A shunt could not be identified, but a bleeding splenic mass is observed when the abdominal cavity is examined.

368. Ovariohysterectomy: The surgery went well, but the polyuria continues.

369. Splenectomy: The spleen is grossly and histologically normal. The dog has a prolonged anesthetic recovery. There is no improvement in the clinical signs.

370. Prednisone administration: The polyuria worsens, the dog begins to eat everything in the house, and the hair on the dog's trunk becomes progressively thinner. Angry clients!

371. Cancer chemotherapy: Chemotherapy alone achieves a short-lived partial remission and the dog survives for another 2 months. If chemotherapy follows a splenectomy, the dog survives for 7 months and the owners are very grateful for your efforts.

372. No treatment: The dog's signs get worse and she begins losing hair on her trunk. The owners take her to another clinic.

373. Adrenalectomy (unilateral): The surgery goes well, but the diarrhea episodes continue and the owners question the need for surgery. They are considering legal action.

374. Cervical vertebral stabilization: The dog develops postoperative vertebral osteomyelitis and the cough continues.

375. Ovariohysterectomy: you cannot find the uterus because the dog is a male; however, you notice a large, bleeding splenic mass.

376. Prednisone administration: There is marked improvement. The dog's cough becomes infrequent, but after the prednisone is tapered down to an every-other-day dose after one month of therapy, the cough begins to increase in frequency.

377. No treatment: The dog's signs progress and it lapses into a coma and dies 2 days later.

378. Cervical vertebral stabilization: There is no improvement in the signs. The dog's signs progress and it lapses into a coma and dies 2 days later.

379. Prednisone administration: The thrombocytopenia gradually resolves over the next 5 days of treatment. The prednisone dosage is gradually reduced over a 4-month period, and the dog experiences no relapses. The owners are thrilled.

380. Bicarbonate administration—parenteral: Although this patient has a metabolic acidosis, it is mild and does not warrant bicarbonate therapy.

381. Fluid therapy—intravenous, replacement type: Mucous membrane pallor, capillary refill time, mental alertness, and strength improve over the next several hours. The dog is stable and doing much better 24 hours later.

382. Thoracocentesis: No pleural fluid was obtained.

383. Thoracocentesis: Approximately 50 ml of fluid was removed from each hemithorax. If this is the only treatment provided, the pleural effusion and dyspnea recur within 1 week.

384. Supplemental oxygen: No response. The dog goes into cardiac arrest 2 hours later and cannot be resuscitated.

385. Pericardiocentesis: You obtain fresh blood because there is no pericardial effusion and you have punctured the heart. The dog goes into cardiac arrest and cannot be resuscitated.

386. Thoracocentesis: No pleural fluid is obtained. The dog goes into cardiac arrest 2 hours later and cannot be resuscitated.

387. Supplemental oxygen: No response. The lethargy and vomiting become worse.

Section VI

Case Summaries and Explanations

Case 1. Episodic weakness in a Doberman pinscher

The main presenting complaint for this dog was episodic weakness. Differential diagnoses that should be considered include:

1. Metabolic abnormalities—e.g., hypokalemia, hyperkalemia, hypercalcemia, hypocalcemia, and hypoglycemia

2. Cardiovascular abnormalities—e.g., arrhythmias, conduction failure, and congestive heart failure

3. Neuromuscular abnormalities—e.g., myasthenia gravis and polymyositis

Based on these considerations, initial diagnostic tests should include a complete blood count, serum biochemical profile, urinalysis, and a neurologic examination. The serum biochemical profile ruled out electrolyte abnormalities and hypoglycemia. The normal creatine kinase (CK) level would also make polymyositis less likely. One could not rule out myasthenia gravis based on a normal neurologic examination. In the absence of an obvious cause for the episodic weakness, assessing the cardiovascular system is indicated. The most appropriate initial tests would be a thoracic radiograph, an electrocardiogram, and a cardiac ultrasound. The presence of a ventricular tachyarrhythmia, and radiographic and echocardiographic signs consistent with dilated cardiomyopathy provide an adequate explanation for the episodic weakness. The periods of weakness were likely caused by paroxysms of ventricular tachycardia. Dilated cardiomyopathy is a common disorder in Doberman pinschers. Further diagnostic testing after this point would be unnecessary. Antiarrhythmic therapy would be indicated and procainamide would be a good first choice for chronic therapy. The dog is not in congestive heart failure, so the administration of furosemide or angiotensin converting enzyme (ACE) inhibitors would not be indicated. The use of digoxin at this stage (compensatory or prefailure) of the disease to enhance myocardial contractility is probably not warranted.

PART

G

Case 2. Acute collapse in a mixed-breed dog

The main presenting complaint was acute collapse. Differential diagnoses that should be considered include:

1. Metabolic abnormalities—e.g., hypokalemia, hyperkalemia, hypercalcemia, hypocalcemia, and hypoglycemia

2. Cardiovascular abnormalities—e.g., arrhythmias, conduction failure, congestive heart failure, and shock

3. Neurologic or neuromuscular abnormalities—e.g., myasthenia gravis and seizures.

Important physical examination findings included pale mucous membranes, a prolonged capillary refill time, tachycardia, and hypothermia, all of which are consistent with a shock state. The major causes of shock are hypovolemia (e.g., blood loss, hypoadrenocorticism), cardiac-related (e.g., heart failure), and diseases that result in distributive (i.e., vasomotor) shock (e.g., sepsis, anaphylaxis). Although a 2/6 systolic murmur was present, there were no other physical signs of heart failure (such as auscultable crackles caused by pulmonary edema, or pulse deficits caused by arrhythmias); this type of murmur is common in middle-aged to older small-breed dogs and is caused by mitral valve endocardiosis. Consequently, this leaves hypovolemia or sepsis as the next most likely cause of the shock. The tense and enlarged abdomen suggests that the cause of the shock might be intra-abdominal, and this should be pursued. Appropriate diagnostic tests would include a complete blood count, serum biochemical profile, urinalysis, abdominal radiograph, abdominocentesis, and abdominal ultrasound. A thoracic radiograph to evaluate the heart and thorax could also be considered. The results of the diagnostic tests suggested intra-abdominal hemorrhage as the cause of the shock, most likely caused by a splenic mass (e.g., hemangiosarcoma). An exploratory laparotomy also would have yielded this information, as long as the dog was stabilized before surgery. Although intra-abdominal hemorrhage caused the shock, the hematocrit was not markedly reduced. Following peracute hemorrhage, the hematocrit will not markedly decrease for several hours, as extracellular fluid moves into the vascular space to compensate, or until intravenous fluids are administered. The mild to moderate thrombocytopenia was likely a consequence of, rather than a cause of, the intra-abdominal hemorrhage. Hemorrhage caused by thrombocytopenia rarely occurs with platelet counts over $20 \times 10^3/\mu l$. Therapeutically, intravenous fluids should be the first treatment. The administration of whole blood would have been acceptable, but the dog may not have required it. Following initial stabilization and the absence of visible metastasis (e.g., normal thoracic radiograph, no evidence on abdominal ultrasound), a splenectomy and possibly postoperative adjunctive chemotherapy could be considered. However, the long-term prognosis for hemangiosarcoma is poor.

Case 3. Epistaxis in a Newfoundland

The main presenting complaint was epistaxis. Differentials that should be considered for a hemorrhagic/bloody nasal discharge include nasal diseases (e.g., trauma, foreign body, neoplasia, fungal infection) and systemic diseases (e.g., coagulopathy, systemic hypertension, polycythemia, vasculitis, hyperviscosity). There was no history of trauma in this dog, and the multiple episodes make trauma an unlikely cause. The relatively acute onset of the hemorrhage (not preceded by sneezing or a serous or mucopurulent nasal discharge) makes neoplasia and fungal infection less likely. On physical examination, petechial hemorrhages were visible on the insides of both pinna and on the oral mucous membranes. This suggests that a coagulopathy may be responsible for the epistaxis. The petechial nature of the hemorrhages also suggests a platelet abnormality as the cause. A complete blood count and serum biochemical profile could be justified to assess the platelet count, hematocrit, and to rule out other systemic disease. This should be done before other more invasive diagnostic tests. The most significant finding was a marked thrombocytopenia, which is the most likely cause of the epistaxis and petechial hemorrhages. The next objective should be to determine the cause of the thrombocytopenia. Differentials for thrombocytopenia include decreased bone marrow production (e.g., infiltrative neoplasia, toxic injury, chronic erhlichiosis), peripheral destruction (e.g., idiopathic immune-mediated, disseminated intravascular coagulation [DIC], acute ehrlichiosis, Rocky Mountain spotted fever [RMSF]), and peripheral sequestration [uncommon] (e.g., splenomegaly, endotoxemia). Serologic testing for ehrlichiosis and Rocky Mountain spotted fever could be justified if the dog resides in a geographic area where these diseases are prevalent (most prevalent in the United States south of the 42nd parallel [ehrlichiosis] and in the eastern United States [RMSF]; very rare in most parts of Canada). In addition, this dog lacks many other signs associated with these rickettsial infections. A bone marrow examination is indicated to rule out decreased marrow production. The results indicated megakaryocytic hyperplasia, and would indicate that peripheral destruction, rather than reduced platelet production, is the cause. In the absence of detectable underlying disease, idiopathic immune-mediated thrombocytopenia is the most likely diagnosis. This is a very common cause of thrombocytopenia in many parts of North America. Prednisone, at immunosuppressive doses, is the initial drug of choice to suppress the immune-mediated destruction. If a urinalysis was performed, mild hematuria would have been detected and was probably caused by the thrombocytopenia. A urine culture was positive, but the low numbers of bacteria cultured would not be considered significant in a free-flow sample, especially in the absence of pyuria.

Case 4. Dyspnea in a domestic shorthaired cat

The main presenting complaint was dyspnea. Differentials that should be considered for the problem of dyspnea include:

1. Upper-airway disease (e.g., laryngeal disease, tracheal obstruction)

2. Lower-airway or pulmonary parenchymal disease (e.g., pneumonia, neoplasia, pulmonary edema)

3. Restrictive or pleural space diseases (e.g., pleural effusion, mediastinal mass, diaphragmatic hernia, pneumothorax)

4. Miscellaneous diseases (e.g.,anemia, heatstroke, neuromuscular weakness)

The physical examination findings of decreased breath sounds and reduced compressibility of the cranial mediastinum would suggest a mediastinal mass, probably accompanied by pleural effusion. Initial diagnostic tests that would be indicated include a complete blood count, serum biochemical profile, and a thoracic radiograph. Further tests could include thoracocentesis (to identify the nature of the pleural fluid), cardiac ultrasound (to rule out cardiac disease and to confirm the presence of a cranial mediastinal mass), and a feline leukemia virus test. The results of these tests indicate a final diagnosis of mediastinal lymphosarcoma, likely caused by feline leukemia virus infection. Although a fine-needle aspirate of the mass could be performed, it is frequently not necessary if pleural fluid can be obtained in cases of lymphosarcoma. These tumors exfoliate large numbers of neoplastic lymphoblasts into the pleural fluid. Therapeutic thoracocentesis to relieve the cat's dyspnea could be considered and would make the cat more comfortable while pursuing other treatments. This cat responded well to chemotherapy, as most cats do, and only transiently to prednisone. Although the longest survival times will be achieved using chemotherapy, the owner must decide whether to use chemotherapy, palliate with prednisone alone, or not to treat at all.

Case 5. Coughing in a miniature dachshund

The main presenting complaint in this dog was coughing. In general, coughing can be caused by one or a combination of the following:

1. Upper-airway disorders (e.g., pharyngitis, collapsing trachea)

2. Lower-airway/pulmonary–parenchymal disorders (e.g., chronic and allergic bronchitis, pneumonia, foreign body)

3. Cardiovascular disorders (e.g., pulmonary edema [i.e., left-sided heart failure], left atrial enlargement, heartworm disease)

The lack of a systolic murmur on physical examination would render both pulmonary edema caused by left-sided heart failure and left atrial enlargement unlikely. Initial diagnostic tests should include a complete blood count and a thoracic radiograph. Eosinophilia and basophilia were present and are caused by type I hypersensitivity (allergic) disorders and parasitism (internal or external). A mild bronchial and interstitial pattern on radiographs suggests lower airway disease, and in combination with the eosinophilia, allergic bronchitis or lungworm infection should be high on the list of differentials. Eosinophila and basophilia can also be present with heartworm infection, and a heartworm antigen test or microfilaria recovery test would certainly be indicated in areas where heartworm infection is a risk. However, the thoracic radiographs did not support heartworm infection (i.e., no pulmonary arterial changes). The next most beneficial diagnostic tests would be a transtracheal wash (to ascertain if there is lower airway disease and whether it is characterized by eosinophilic inflammation) and fecal examinations (routine flotation and a Baermann examination to detect parasitic infection that may be pulmonary [e.g., lungworm]). The results of these tests indicated that eosinophilic airway inflammation was indeed present, and the Baermann fecal examination revealed a lungworm infection (in this case, *Crenosoma vulpis*—a fox lungworm). If the fecal examinations were negative, a diagnosis of allergic bronchitis would have been justified. The most appropriate treatment would be fenbendazole. This anthelmintic is effective against most lungworm infections in dogs.

Case 6. Depression and ataxia in a mixed-breed dog

The main presenting problems in this case were mental depression, ataxia, cervical pain, and slow pupillary light reflexes. The cervical pain and neurologic examination findings consistent with a C1 to C5 lesion would be compatible with meningitis (bacterial, fungal, nonseptic), disk disease, vertebral fracture/luxation, vertebral neoplasia, and diskospondylitis. The mental depression would indicate a lesion in the rostral midbrain or cerebral cortex. This finding, along with signs suggestive of a C1–C5 lesion, would suggest multifocal or diffuse central nervous system (CNS) disease caused by inflammatory/infectious etiologies or metastatic neoplasia. Neoplasia would be less likely because of the dog's young age. The slow pupillary light reflexes should have prompted a fundoscopic examination, which would reveal retinal detachment and chorioretinitis. Differentials for this finding could include fungal infection, canine distemper virus, granulomatous meningoencephalitis, lymphosarcoma, ehrlichiosis, and Rocky Mountain spotted fever (plus others). Due to the systemic signs of illness, a complete blood count, serum biochemical profile, and urinalysis were indicated, but were all normal. Given these findings and differentials, cerebrospinal fluid collection would be the next logical diagnostic test. The results indicated CNS cryptococcosis. Although not required to make the diagnosis in this case, a cryptococcal capsular antigen test (serum) was positive. Antifungal drug treatment would be indicated, but the efficacy varies among the antifungal agents. Fluconazole is probably the best choice because it penetrates into the CNS better than any other agent. Ketoconazole or amphotericin B may be effective but an incomplete response or a relapse would be more common with these agents. Regardless of the antifungal agent chosen, the prognosis for a long-term cure of CNS cryptococcosis is guarded.

Case 7. Increased urination in a miniature poodle

The main presenting complaint for this dog was increased urination. Based on the history of increased urine volume and probable increased water consumption, the problem can be further defined as polyuria. Differential diagnoses that should be considered include iatrogenic causes (e.g., medications, low-protein diet), central diabetes insipidus, diabetes mellitus,

Escherichia coli infection, hepatic disease, hyperadrenocorticism, hypercalcemia, hyperthyroidism, hypoadrenocorticism, hypokalemia, nephrogenic diabetes insipidus (congenital or secondary), polycythemia, pyelonephritis, pyometra, renal failure, renal glucosuria, and psychogenic polydipsia. Based on these considerations, initial diagnostic tests would include a complete blood count, serum biochemical profile, urinalysis, and possible abdominal radiographs and serum osmolality. The history eliminated iatrogenic causes. The complete blood count ruled out polycythemia. The serum biochemical profile ruled out diabetes mellitus, hypercalcemia, and hypokalemia, and made significant renal failure unlikely. The markedly increased serum alkaline phosphatase (ALP) concentration made hyperadrenocorticism a strong possibility, although cholestasis can also increase ALP. On the urinalysis, the urine specific gravity was consistent with polyuria. Renal glucosuria and diabetes mellitus were eliminated from the list of differential diagnoses based on the lack of glucosuria, and a urinary tract infection was identified. If abdominal radiographs were obtained, the identified hepatomegaly would also support possible hyperadrenocorticism. Serum osmolality was not helpful. Based on the initial test results and the clinical signs, hyperadrenocorticism and a urinary tract infection seemed most likely. A screening test for hyperadrenocorticism should be performed, and a urine culture should be submitted. Either an adrenocorticotropic hormone (ACTH) stimulation test or low-dose dexamethasone suppression test would yield a diagnosis of hyperadrenocorticism in this dog; results of a urine cortisol:creatinine ratio do not rule out hyperadrenocorticism, but do not confirm it either. Once hyperadrenocorticism is identified, a high-dose dexamethasone suppression test, an endogenous basal ACTH concentration, abdominal (adrenal) ultrasound, or results of the low-dose dexamethasone suppression test will further define the problem as pituitary-dependent hyperadrenocorticism in this dog. Computerized tomography of the abdomen (adrenals) will also allow this differentiation, but is more costly and less widely available. Results of the urine culture confirm the presence of a urinary tract infection.

The hyperadrenocorticism can be treated with mitotane (o'p-DDD), ketoconazole, or bilateral adrenalectomy, although the latter has significantly greater risks and requires subsequent lifelong treatment of the patient for hypoadrenocorticism. Cephalexin or ampicillin is a good choice for treatment of the urinary tract infection.

Case 8. Increased urination and hematuria in a German shepherd

The main presenting complaints for this dog were increased urination and possible hematuria. Based on the history of frequent urination of small amounts, the increased urination could be further defined as pollakiuria. Differential diagnoses for pollakiuria would include urinary tract infection, cystic calculi, bladder or urethral neoplasia, or urethral spasm. In a male dog, prostatic disease should also be considered. Differential diagnoses for hematuria would include urinary tract infection, cystic calculi, urinary tract neoplasia, coagulopathies, and idiopathic renal hematuria; because of the concurrent pollakiuria, coagulopathies or idiopathic renal hematuria are less likely. Based on these considerations, initial diagnostic tests would include a complete blood count, urinalysis, and possible serum biochemical profile and abdominal radiographs. The urinalysis confirms the hematuria, but there is not concurrent leukuria or crystalluria; the urine specific gravity rules out polyuria as a component of the problem. A serum biochemical profile does not narrow the list of possible diagnoses, but does rule out significant concurrent renal failure. Abdominal radiographs rule out radiodense cystic calculi. A urine culture will rule out urinary tract infection. Based on the remaining differential diagnoses, abdominal (bladder and prostate) ultrasound and/or a contrast cystogram should be performed next. Either procedure identifies a probable mass in the trigone area of the bladder. Based on the location and the most common types of bladder tumors, this is most likely a transitional cell carcinoma, but a biopsy is required for definitive diagnosis. If the tumor is small, surgical resection can be attempted, but this is rarely possible because of the proximity, and often intimate involvement, of the mass with the ureters and the urethra. Chemotherapy may result in partial remission or slow the progression of the disease but is not curative.

Case 9. Intermittent diarrhea in a mixed-breed dog

The main presenting complaint for this dog was chronic intermittent diarrhea. The diarrhea is probably of both small and large bowel origin, based respectively on the history of weight loss and occasional fresh blood in the feces. Differential diagnoses for chronic or intermittent small bowel diarrhea that should be considered include both extra-gastrointestinal disorders (e.g., exocrine pancreatic insufficiency, hepatic disease, hypoadrenocorticism, chronic pancreatitis, renal disease) and primary gastrointestinal disorders (e.g., dietary intolerance, infection [bacterial, fungal], inflammatory bowel disease, irritable bowel syndrome, lymphangiectasia, neoplasia, partial mechanical obstruction, physiologic obstruction, parasites, small intestinal bacterial overgrowth, villous atrophy). Exocrine pancreatic insufficiency, hepatic disease, renal disease, infection, lymphangiectasia, neoplasia, partial obstruction, small intestinal bacterial overgrowth, and villous atrophy would be less likely because the diarrhea is intermittent in this dog and these disorders tend to cause more persistent diarrhea. Differential diagnoses for chronic or intermittent large bowel diarrhea include dietary intolerance, infection (algal, bacterial, fungal), inflammatory colitis, neoplasia, partial obstruction, parasites, and stress colitis/irritable colon. Again, infection, neoplasia, and a partial obstruction would be less likely because the diarrhea in this dog is intermittent and these disorders tend to cause more persistent diarrhea. Based on these considerations, initial diagnostic tests would include a complete blood count, serum biochemical profile, urinalysis, fecal examinations for parasites, and abdominal radiographs. Negative fecal examinations and the prior deworming with fenbendazole rule out most parasites. The serum biochemical profile rules out renal disease, most hepatic disease, and typical hypoadrenocorticism, although 'atypical' hypoadrenocorticism (i.e., just glucocorticoid deficiency) could not be eliminated. The presence of panhypoproteinemia in the absence of proteinuria suggests a protein-losing enteropathy and primary intestinal disease. Because of this, further diagnostic testing should be aimed at the intestinal tract. Gastrointestinal function tests (e.g., serum cobalamin and folate concentrations, fat absorption test) would not be inappropriate but are not needed to identify the intestine as the site of disease. At this point, endoscopic or surgical intestinal biopsies are indicated. Biopsies yield a diagnosis of inflammatory bowel disease (i.e., lymphocytic-plasmacytic enterocolitis). Treatment with a low-fat, highly digestible diet, a "hypoallergenic" diet, metronidazole, prednisone, or a combination of these treatments usually controls the disease.

Case 10. Anorexia and weakness in a Great Dane

The major problems identified in this dog were circulatory shock (weak pulses, prolonged capillary refill time [CRT], and weakness) and bradycardia. Differential diagnoses that should be considered for shock include fluid loss (e.g., blood, gastrointestinal [GI] fluid losses), sepsis, hypoadrenocorticism, and cardiac failure. There was no history of hemorrhage, gastrointestinal fluid loss, trauma, or toxin exposure. Differential diagnoses that should be considered for bradycardia include primary cardiac disease, electrolyte imbalances, increased vagal tone, or central nervous system disease. Toxicity, hypothermia, or drug-induced bradycardia were unlikely. Weakness, if not secondary to shock, could also have been due to:

1. Neuromuscular disease (e.g., myopathies, junctionopathies, neuropathies, myelopathies, spinal cord disease or compression)

2. Cardiovascular disease (e.g., congenital defects, arrhythmias, dirofilariasis, myocardial disease, bacterial endocarditis, pericardial disease, neoplasia)

3. Metabolic disease (e.g., hypoglycemia, hepatic encephalopathy, hypercalcemia, hypocalcemia, hyperkalemia, hypokalemia, anemia)

A metabolic or cardiovascular cause of weakness should be considered most likely based on the concurrent shock and bradycardia.

Based on these considerations, initial diagnostic tests should include a complete blood count, serum biochemical profile, urinalysis, thoracic radiographs, and an electrocardiogram. The microcardia found on thoracic radiographs supported the clinical suspicion of hypovolemia. The electrocardiographic changes were consistent with hyperkalemia. The serum biochemical profile confirmed severe hyperkalemia and revealed mild hyponatremia, mild hypochloremia, and azotemia. The urine was not concentrated despite the clinical dehydration and azotemia. These results were most consistent with hypoadrenocorticism or acute renal failure.

This is an extremely ill dog requiring prompt and aggressive emergency treatment. The hyperkalemia in this patient is life-threatening and must be treated immediately; saline diuresis, glucose and/or insulin administration, or bicarbonate administration could be used to lower the serum potassium concentration. Calcium gluconate administration could also be useful for its cardioprotective effects. Intravenous fluid administration, either saline or other replacement fluid, is also needed as treatment for the shock.

Immediately following, or in conjunction with treatment of the hyperkalemia, an adrenocorticotropic hormone (ACTH) stimulation test should be performed to differentiate hypoadrenocorticism from acute renal failure. If prednisone was administered prior to this test, the results would be invalid because the assay will detect the administered prednisone as cortisol. Dexamethasone does not cross-react with the cortisol assay and is the glucocorticoid of choice in the patient with suspected hypoadrenocorticism where an ACTH stimulation test is planned. The ACTH stimulation test results in this dog confirmed a diagnosis of hypoadrenocorticism, indicating a need for long-term management with fludrocortisone with or without additional low-dose prednisone therapy. With appropriate treatment, the long-term prognosis is excellent.

Case 11. Seizures in a miniature schnauzer

The main presenting complaint for this dog was seizures. Differential diagnoses that should be considered include both extracranial disorders (e.g., hypoglycemia, hypocalcemia, hepatic encephalopathy, uremia, hypoxia, and toxins) and intracranial disorders (e.g., infection, inflammation, congenital disorders, neoplasia, idiopathic epilepsy). Based on these considerations, initial diagnostic tests should include a complete blood count, serum biochemical profile, and urinalysis. The biochemical profile ruled out hypocalcemia and uremia and made hypoglycemia less likely. Hypoalbuminemia in the absence of proteinuria, a low normal glucose concentration, and a low normal cholesterol concentration are suggestive of hepatic dysfunction with decreased hepatic production of these substances.

Based on these considerations, a liver function test (e.g., serum bile acid concentrations, blood ammonia) and abdominal radiographs should be performed next. The function tests confirmed severe hepatic dysfunction and radiographs showed microhepatica. In a young dog, these results are most consistent with a probable portosystemic shunt. Ultrasound will sometimes identify the aberrant vessel(s) but a contrast portogram or rectal portal scintigraphy (not available in the diagnostic test list) are more consistent methods of shunt identification. A splenoportogram identified a single extrahepatic shunt in this dog. Surgical ligation of the shunt is the optimal means of treatment. Medical treatment (i.e., reduced protein diet, oral lactulose, oral neomycin) can be helpful preoperatively or in patients with an inoperable shunt. Emergency treatment of acute severe signs of hepatic encephalopathy may also include intravenous fluid administration, correction of electrolyte imbalances or hypoglycemia, and administration of lactulose enemas. Cystic uroliths, most likely ammonium urate, were also identified in this patient. Surgical removal at the time of shunt closure is the usual treatment, although dietary dissolution could be considered.

Case 12. Vomiting and lethargy in a golden retriever

The main presenting complaints for this dog were vomiting and lethargy. Differential diagnoses for the vomiting that should be considered include both extragastrointestinal disorders (e.g., central nervous system disease, diabetic ketoacidosis, hepatic disease, hypercalcemia, hypo-adrenocorticism, hypocalcemia, hypokalemia, pancreatitis, peritonitis, pyometra, renal disease, sepsis, urinary obstruction) and primary gastrointestinal disorders (e.g., gastric dilation, gastritis/enteritis, gastric or upper intestinal obstruction, neoplasia, obstipation, ulcers, toxins). Based on these differentials, initial diagnostic tests should include a complete blood count, serum biochemical profile, urinalysis, and abdominal radiographs. The complete blood count showed an inflammatory leukogram with a shift toward immaturity consistent with an infectious or inflammatory disorder. The biochemical profile ruled out diabetes mellitus, hypercalcemia, typical hypoadrenocorticism, hypocalcemia, hypokalemia, and renal disease and made pancreatitis unlikely. The radiographic findings of a large tubular structure in the mid-caudal abdomen in conjunction with the history of recent estrus in this dog make a closed-cervix pyometra the most likely diagnosis. Abdominal ultrasound confirms the diagnosis if pregnancy is also a possible cause of the enlarged uterus.

Treatment requires intravenous fluids to correct the dehydration, antibiotic therapy and removal of the uterus or evacuation of the uterine contents. With a closed-cervix pyometra, ovariohysterectomy is the optimal treatment; most dogs recovery very quickly following removal of the infected organ. If the dog's primary use is as a breeding animal, use of prostaglandin $F_{2\alpha}$ to cause contraction of the uterus and expulsion of the infected contents can be considered, but with a closed-cervix pyometra this carries an increased risk of uterine rupture. Prostaglandin therapy is also not recommended for treatment of pyometra in a dog with systemic signs of illness because the treatment does not eliminate the infection as quickly as ovariohysterectomy.

3521243